Handbook
of Nonprescription
Drugs Quick Reference

Handbook
of Nonprescription
Drugs Quick Reference

Cortney M. Mospan, PharmD, BCACP, BCGP
Co-Editor
Assistant Professor of Pharmacy
Wingate University School of Pharmacy

Miranda Wilhelm, PharmD
Co-Editor
Clinical Associate Professor of Pharmacy Practice
Southern Illinois University Edwardsville School
of Pharmacy

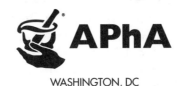

APhA

WASHINGTON, DC

Acquisition Editor: Janan Sarwar
Managing Editors: John Fedor and Janan Sarwar
Composition Services: Circle Graphics
Cover Design: Michelle Powell, APhA Integrated Design and Production Center
Editorial Services: J&J Editorial LLC

Published by the American Pharmacists Association
2215 Constitution Avenue, NW
Washington, DC 29937-2985
www.pharmacist.com www.pharmacylibrary.com

To comment on this book via e-mail, send your message to the publisher at aphabooks@aphanet.org.

Library of Congress Cataloguing-in-Publication Data

Names: Mospan, Cortney M. editor. | Wilhelm, Miranda, editor. | American
   Pharmacists Association, issuing body.
Title: Handbook of nonprescription drugs quick reference / Cortney M. Mospan,
   Miranda Wilhelm, co-editors.
Other titles: Digest of (work): Handbook of nonprescription drugs.
Description: Washington, DC : American Pharmacists Association, [2019] |
   Digest of Handbook of nonprescription drugs : an interactive approach to
   self-care / editor-in-chief: Daniel L. Krinsky. 19th edition. 2018. |
   Includes bibliographical references.
Identifiers: LCCN 2019005691 | ISBN 9781582122908
Subjects: | MESH: Nonprescription Drugs | Handbook
Classification: LCC RM671.A1 | NLM QV 39 | DDC 615.1--dc23 LC record available
at https://lccn.loc.gov/2019005691

Contents

Preface

This book is intended to be a resource for busy practitioners and students when approached by a patient for a self-care recommendation. It is designed to be used in the aisle to enable practitioners to use the text to determine if patients are candidates for self-care. Once the patient is determined to have a self-treatable condition, this tool assists practitioners in real time to confidently make a self-care treatment recommendation. Each chapter is organized to help practitioners identify the optimal treatment based on the condition and bothersome symptom(s), enhancing efficiency in the self-care process.

The chapters and appendices in this book address common self-treatable conditions for which patients seek treatment recommendations. Each chapter begins with an algorithm to determine if the patient is a candidate for self-care. Within each chapter, the treatment approach is organized using the QuEST SCHOLAR MAC format, helping practitioners walk through this standardized process for self-care assessment for each condition. The first chapter of the book provides an extensive review of the QuEST SCHOLAR process and how it can improve self-care treatment recommendations. Special highlights of this text include sample assessment questions using the SCHOLAR acronym, considerations for special populations, patient counseling recommendations, clinical pearls, and a concise summary of appropriate nonprescription medication recommendations for each condition.

This book is intended to be complementary to the more detailed *Handbook of Nonprescription Drugs*, and practitioners are encouraged to consult the *Handbook of Nonprescription Drugs* for a thorough review of information about the conditions covered in this book. The *Handbook of Nonprescription Drugs* also contains content for a number of conditions that are not covered in this book. The *Nonprescription Drugs Quick Reference* chapters were developed using content from the *Handbook of Nonprescription Drugs: An Interactive Approach to Self-Care*, 19th edition. The information has been edited and formatted to include only content that practitioners are most likely to need during self-care consultations with patients and has been reformatted in organization and flow to better match the patient assessment process in practice.

In addition, practitioners should consult the Drug Facts label of all nonprescription products they recommend to verify the active ingredient(s), dosages, and instructions for use. We hope this is a useful tool for you to make safe, effective, and appropriate nonprescription recommendations for self-care conditions.

Cortney M. Mospan, PharmD, BCACP, BCGP
Co-Editor
Assistant Professor of Pharmacy
Wingate University School of Pharmacy

Miranda Wilhelm, PharmD
Co-Editor
Clinical Associate Professor
Southern Illinois University Edwardsville School of Pharmacy

Editors of the *Handbook of Nonprescription Drugs: An Interactive Approach to Self-Care*, 19th Edition

Editor-in-Chief
Daniel L. Krinsky, MS, RPh

Associate Editors
Stefanie P. Ferreri, PharmD, CDE, FAPhA
Brian A. Hemstreet, PharmD, FCCP, BCPS
Anne Lamont Hume, PharmD, FCCP, BCPS
Gail D. Newton, PhD, RPh
Carol J. Rollins, MS, RD, PharmD, BCNSP
Karen J. Tietze, PharmD

Contributors

Erin N. Adams, PharmD, BCACP
Associate Professor of Pharmacy Practice
Bernard J. Dunn School of Pharmacy
Shenandoah University — Fairfax Campus
Fairfax, Virginia

Nabila Ahmed-Sarwar, PharmD, BCPS, BCACP, CDE, BC-ADM
Associate Professor of Pharmacy Practice
St. John Fisher College, Wegman's School of Pharmacy
Rochester, New York

Albert Bach, PharmD
Assistant Professor of Pharmacy Practice
Chapman University School of Pharmacy
Irvine, California

Cynthia Knapp Dlugosz, BSPharm
Owner, CKD Associates LLC
Ann Arbor, Michigan

Connie Kang, PharmD, BCPS, BCGP
Assistant Professor of Clinical Sciences
Keck Graduate Institute School of Pharmacy and Health Sciences
Claremont, California

Cortney M. Mospan, PharmD, BCACP, BCGP
Assistant Professor of Pharmacy
Wingate University School of Pharmacy
Wingate, North Carolina

Karen Steinmetz Pater, PharmD, CDE, BCACP
Associate Professor, Department of Pharmacy and Therapeutics
University of Pittsburgh School of Pharmacy
Pittsburgh, Pennsylvania

Rashi Chandra Waghel, PharmD, BCACP
Associate Professor of Pharmacy
Wingate University School of Pharmacy
Wingate, North Carolina

Miranda Wilhelm, PharmD
Clinical Associate Professor of Pharmacy Practice
Southern Illinois University Edwardsville School of Pharmacy
Edwardsville, Illinois

Jennifer A. Wilson, PharmD, BCACP
Associate Professor of Pharmacy
Wingate University School of Pharmacy
Wingate, North Carolina

The "QuEST" Approach to Self-Care Encounters

Cynthia Knapp Dlugosz, BSPharm

According to Consumer Healthcare Products Association data, more than 80% of adults in the United States use over-the-counter (OTC) products as a first response to minor ailments.[1] Ideally, patients make informed choices about self-care, increasing the likelihood that they will use effective therapies and lessening the chance that they will engage in unsafe self-treatment.

Pharmacists are the logical health care professionals to assist patients (or their caregivers or proxies) with self-care decisions. Pharmacists often are available at the point of purchase of OTC products. They also are the only health care professionals who receive in-depth formal education and skill development in nonprescription pharmacotherapy.

When pharmacists assist with patients' self-care needs, they must perform functions usually performed by a patient's primary care provider: assess the patient, formulate a presumptive diagnosis, and recommend a treatment option based on the subjective (and sometimes objective) information available. Specifically, pharmacists need to

- gather and evaluate information about the patient's problem or symptom(s) and overall health status;

- differentiate self-treatable conditions from conditions that require medical intervention;

- advise and counsel the patient about the best course of action. Examples of possible courses of action are (1) no treatment, (2) self-treatment with nonprescription medications or nondrug measures, and (3) referral to a primary care provider or other health care provider.

The "QuEST" process was designed to help pharmacists identify a self-treating patient's chief complaints and recommend an efficacious treatment approach in a time-efficient manner. As shown in Table 1, QuEST stands for

- **Qu**ickly and accurately assess the patient;

- **E**stablish that the patient is an appropriate self-care candidate;

- **S**uggest appropriate self-care strategies to the patient;

- **T**alk with the patient about the selected self-care strategies.

The QuEST process was created in 2001 by three health care communications experts (Kenneth Leibowitz, MA; Helen Meldrum, EdD; and Diane Ginsburg, MS) as part of an American Pharmacists Association (APhA) continuing education training program. It subsequently was presented at the inaugural APhA Self-Care Institute in 2002.

TABLE 1. The QuEST process

Quickly and accurately assess the patient (using SCHOLAR-MAC)

- Ask about current complaint (SCHOLAR)
- Ask about medications and other products (M)
- Ask about allergies to medications (A)
- Ask about coexisting conditions (C)

Establish that the patient is an appropriate self-care candidate

- No severe symptoms
- No symptoms that persist or return repeatedly
- No self-treating to avoid medical care

Suggest appropriate self-care strategies to the patient

- Medication
- Alternative therapies
- General care measures

Talk with the patient about the selected self-care strategies

- Counsel on medication actions, administration, and adverse effects
- Describe what to expect from treatment
- Discuss appropriate follow-up

■ ■ Quickly and Accurately Assess the Patient

The first step in the QuEST process is to assess the patient as quickly and accurately as possible. Note the deliberate use of the word *quickly*. Pharmacists should focus on collecting the information that will be of greatest use: (1) details about the patient's current problem; (2) any concurrent medications; (3) known allergies or sensitivities to medications; and (4) coexisting conditions or disease states.

The acronym "SCHOLAR" is a mnemonic for the types of information that help to ensure a thorough characterization of the patient's current problem. The acronym "MAC" reminds pharmacists to ask about medications, allergies, and coexisting conditions.

■ *Information About the Current Problem*

The patient interview begins with an exploration of the patient's chief complaint. Table 2 lists the components of SCHOLAR and provides examples of questions that can elicit the various types of information.

SCHOLAR is not an algorithm that must be followed step by step. Pharmacists should use professional judgment and common sense when asking the SCHOLAR questions. Not all of these questions need to be asked of all patients, and the questions may not need to be asked in the specific order presented.

TABLE 2. SCHOLAR mnemonic for characterizing a patient's current problem

Symptoms
- What is bothering you?
- What is wrong?
- What other problems (or symptoms) have you noticed?

Characteristics of the symptoms or problem, Course of the symptoms or problem
- What does the pain (or problem) feel like?
- Describe your symptoms (or problem).
- How are your symptoms changing over time (better, worse, same)?
- How bothersome are your symptoms?
- To what extent do your symptoms interfere with your usual or desired activities (e.g., sleeping, eating, working, walking)?

History of symptoms in past
- When have you suffered from the same symptoms or similar symptoms in the past?
- How has this problem (or these symptoms) affected you in the past?
- What have you done (or what has been done) in the past to alleviate the problem or symptoms? What were the results?

Onset
- When did this problem (or these symptoms) start?
- How often do the symptoms occur?
- How did the problem (or symptoms) start?
- What were you doing when you first noticed the symptoms?
- How long have the symptoms been present? How long have you had this problem?

Location
- Where does it hurt?
- Where is the problem located?
- In what part of your body are you experiencing symptoms?

Aggravating factors
- What (food, medication, activity, position) makes the problem (or symptoms) worse?
- What else do you feel when you have this problem?

Relieving factors
- What (food, medication, activity, position) makes the problem (or symptoms) better?
- What have you done so far to make the problem better (or relieve the symptoms), and was it successful?

Source: Adapted from Wheeler SQ, Windt JH. *Telephone Triage: Theory, Practice, and Protocol Development.* Albany, NY: Delmar Publishers; 1993.

When asking patients about their chief complaint, it is important not to confuse the patient's self-diagnosis with the patient's symptoms. The patient's self-diagnosis may not be correct, so pharmacists always should form an independent assessment based on the information they collect. Pharmacists should refrain from implying acceptance of the patient's theory; instead, they should simply acknowledge the patient's theory and then proceed with the interview. For example, if the patient were to say to the pharmacist:

"I don't know what's wrong. I think I have the flu, but it's lasted so long and I've tried everything. It's been going on now for 2 weeks."

The pharmacist might respond:

"Well, some people who get the flu do feel sick for quite some time, but I'm not sure that what you have is the flu. What symptoms have you noticed?"

The SCHOLAR components assume that the pharmacist is interacting directly with the patient. When the pharmacist interacts with the patient's caregiver or representative (e.g., the parent of a young child, the patient's husband or wife), the pharmacist should ask additional questions to learn about the patient, such as:

- How old is the patient? If the patient is a child, how much does the patient weigh?

- Is the patient male or female? If the patient is a female, is she pregnant or breastfeeding?

Information About Medications

The second part of the patient interview involves obtaining as complete a list as possible of the prescription medications, nonprescription medications, herbal products, and dietary supplements that the patient is using, as well as the problems or conditions for which the patient is using them. It also is helpful to know about the patient's use of alcohol, caffeine, tobacco, and recreational drugs, because this information may influence the pharmacist's evaluation of whether the patient is a suitable candidate for self-treatment (e.g., a cough in a patient who smokes may need to be evaluated by a physician) or the eventual self-treatment recommendation (e.g., the need to warn a patient about concurrent use of alcohol and pain relievers). The pharmacist should take care to explain why this information is necessary and phrase queries in a nonjudgmental manner. For example, "Some medications can interact with alcoholic beverages. To help me determine the best medication for you, please tell me about your usual consumption of beer, wine, or liquor."

Information About Allergies

In addition to finding out which medications and products a patient uses regularly, pharmacists should inquire whether the patient is allergic to any medications or products. Keep in mind that patients might not differentiate true allergic reactions from sensitivities and adverse effects (e.g., stomach upset from aspirin).

⬛ Information About Coexisting Conditions

Information about coexisting conditions is needed to avoid possible drug–disease interactions, as well as to establish that the patient is an appropriate candidate for self-treatment. Some of this information will come from the medication history. Examples of questions that help to elicit additional information include:

- For what other types of problems or conditions do you routinely see your doctor?

- What other illnesses have been acting up lately?

- What other problems do you have with your health?

⬛⬛ Establish That the Patient Is an Appropriate Self-Care Candidate

The information pharmacists gather during the assessment step helps in formulating a presumptive diagnosis and determining whether the patient is an appropriate candidate for self-care. Patients who are not appropriate self-care candidates should be referred to a primary care provider. In general, referral is indicated in the following situations:

- The patient's symptoms are too severe to be endured without definitive diagnosis and treatment.

- The symptoms are minor but persistent and do not appear to be the result of an easily identifiable cause.

- The symptoms have recurred repeatedly with no recognizable cause.

- The patient has symptom-specific exclusions to self-treatment.

- The pharmacist is in doubt about the patient's medical condition.

The pharmacist should be precise about where and when the treatment should take place. Does the patient require care within minutes, hours, or days? Should the patient be evaluated in an emergency department, urgent care clinic, or physician's office? Patients with emergent, urgent, or semiurgent symptoms should be given specific instructions to avoid confusion and decrease possible patient denial. For example:

- "You must be seen by a physician within 2 hours. Are you able to get to the emergency department within 2 hours, or should we call an ambulance?"

- "Call your physician's office as soon as you get home to arrange an appointment. Ask for an appointment this afternoon, or no later than tomorrow morning."

■ ■ Suggest Appropriate Self-Care Strategies to the Patient

If the patient does appear to be a candidate for self-treatment, the pharmacist must collaborate with the patient to select an appropriate treatment strategy based on the pharmacist's presumptive diagnosis of the patient's condition. If self-treatment with a nonprescription product is indicated, the pharmacist may need to ask additional questions at this point to assist with product selection. For example, can the patient swallow a solid dosage form? Must the patient stay alert? If the patient asks about options such as herbal products, the pharmacist should provide information—as evidence-based as possible—about the relative merits and drawbacks of the product in an unbiased and nonjudgmental manner.

■ ■ Talk With the Patient About the Selected Self-Care Strategies

The final step in the self-care encounter is to discuss the recommended course of action with the patient. If self-treatment with a nonprescription product is indicated, the pharmacist should counsel the patient about the topics listed in Table 3. Ideally, pharmacists should accompany patients to the appropriate aisle, select the appropriate product from the shelf, and point out important information on the Drug Facts label. Providing patients with supplemental written information when necessary also can help to ensure that instructions are followed accurately.

As part of counseling, pharmacists should explain what the patient should expect during the next few hours or days, both in the normal course of the condition and subsequent to treatment measures. Patients should understand the symptoms or developments that indicate failure of self-treatment or possible complications. Whenever possible, pharmacists should follow up with self-treating patients to

TABLE 3. Counseling points for self-treating patients

- The reasons for self-treatment
- Description of the medication or treatment
  - Name
  - Mechanism of action
  - Expected effect
- Proper administration of the medication or treatment
  - Dose and dosage schedule
  - Route of administration
  - Duration of therapy
- What to expect from treatment
- How soon to expect results
- Precautions
- Anticipated adverse effects and how to manage them
- General treatment guidelines
- Appropriate follow-up
- Other important information (e.g., storage requirements)

- determine whether the condition was managed successfully with the self-treatment recommendations;

- find out whether the patient sought medical evaluation as recommended;

- inquire whether any new symptoms had emerged;

- provide advice about managing any adverse effects.

Follow-up could occur formally (e.g., by setting up a future appointment) or informally (e.g., a telephone call inquiring how the patient is doing). However, not all patients will be receptive to follow-up encounters. One strategy is to conclude each self-care encounter by presenting patients with a business card and offering to follow up with them in an appropriate number of days. That way, patients who decline the offer for follow-up still would have the pharmacist's contact information in the event that any new problems or questions were to arise.

⬛ ⬤ References

1. Consumer Healthcare Products Association. Statistics on OTC use. http://www.chpa.org/MarketStats.aspx. Accessed February 15, 2016.

QuEST/SCHOLAR-MAC at a Glance

The QuEST Process

Qu ickly and accurately assess the patient (SCHOLAR-MAC)

- Ask about current complaint (SCHOLAR)
- Ask about medications and other products (M)
- Ask about allergies (A)
- Ask about coexisting conditions (C)

E stablish that the patient is an appropriate self-care candidate

- No severe symptoms
- No symptoms that persist or return repeatedly
- No self-treating to avoid medical care

S uggest appropriate self-care strategies

- Medication
- Alternative treatments
- General care measures

T alk with the patient

- Counsel on medication actions, administration, and adverse effects
- Describe what to expect from treatment
- Discuss appropriate follow-up

SCHOLAR

S ymptoms

- What are the main and associated symptoms?

C haracteristics

- What is the situation like? Is it changing?

H istory

- What has been done so far?

O nset

- When did it start?

L ocation

- Where is the problem?

A ggravating factors

- What makes it worse?

R emitting factors

- What makes it better?

MAC

M edications

A llergies

C oexisting conditions

ACNE

Nabila Ahmed-Sarwar, PharmD, BCPS, BCACP, CDE, BC-ADM

For complete information about this topic, consult Chapter 38, "Acne," written by Karla T. Foster and published in the *Handbook of Nonprescription Drugs*, 19th Edition.[1]

Self-Care of Acne

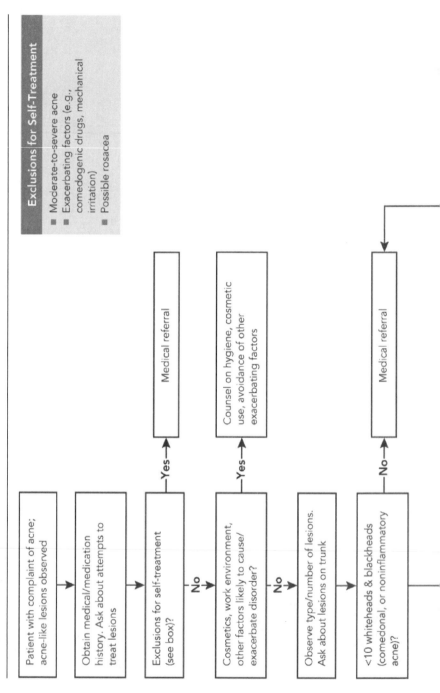

Exclusions for Self-Treatment

- Moderate-to-severe acne
- Exacerbating factors (e.g., comedogenic drugs, mechanical irritation)
- Possible rosacea

Patient with complaint of acne; acne-like lesions observed

Obtain medical/medication history. Ask about attempts to treat lesions

Exclusions for self-treatment (see box)? —Yes→ Medical referral

No

Cosmetics, work environment, other factors likely to cause/ exacerbate disorder? —Yes→ Counsel on hygiene, cosmetic use, avoidance of other exacerbating factors

No

Observe type/number of lesions. Ask about lesions on trunk

<10 whiteheads & blackheads (comedonal, or noninflammatory acne)? —No→ Medical referral

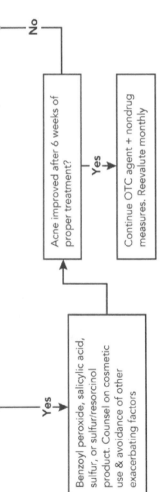

Yes

Benzoyl peroxide, salicylic acid, sulfur, or sulfur/resorcinol product. Counsel on cosmetic use & avoidance of other exacerbating factors

Acne improved after 6 weeks of proper treatment?

No

Yes

Continue OTC agent + nondrug measures. Reevaluate monthly

OTC = over-the-counter.

■■ Overview

■ Acne vulgaris (AV), or acne, is an inflammatory skin disease. Acne lesions most commonly occur on the face but also may be found on the back, chest, shoulders, and neck.

■ Acne is a self-limiting condition that can persist for long periods, requiring continuous and consistent treatment. There is no cure for acne.

■ The goals of self-treatment are to reduce symptoms and minimize scarring.

■■ Pathophysiology

■ The pilosebaceous unit located in the dermis of the skin is home to the sebaceous gland, which acts as an endocrine organ and is responsible for sebum production. Sebum is a skin protectant and possesses antibacterial properties that mediate inflammation and support wound healing.

■ The development of acne involves four major factors; these include increased sebum production, follicular colonization of *Propionibacterium acnes (P. acnes)*, follicular hyperkeratinization, and an increase in inflammatory mediator release in the skin.

■ An increase in androgen production in the adolescent years increases sebum production and alters follicular desquamation. Early lesion formation may be stimulated by the release of inflammatory mediators from follicular keratinocytes as the lesion develops excessive sebum, which serves as a growth medium for *P. acnes*.

■■ QuEST: Quickly and Accurate Assess the Patient Using SCHOLAR MAC

QuEST SCHOLAR is an acronym used to assess a patient to determine self-care candidate status and identify which treatment would be most appropriate. See Chapter 1 for a description of the QuEST SCHOLAR process.

■ Does the Patient Have Acne?

■ Acne is indicated by the presence of a combination of inflammatory and noninflammatory acne lesions on the face, chest, or back. Occasionally, lesions may appear on the neck or upper arms.

- Noninflammatory lesions include open (blackheads) or closed (whiteheads) comedones.

- Inflammatory lesions are small prominent inflamed elevations in the skin, which are referred to as pimples or papules. Pustules result from papules becoming enlarged and pus filled.

- A number of factors are known to exacerbate existing acne and cause periodic flare-ups of acne in some patients. See Table 1 for exacerbating factors in acne.

● *Important SCHOLAR MAC Considerations*

- What is the patient's age?
  - Onset coincides with changes in androgen levels. Acne is most prevalent in girls between the ages of 14-17 years and boys between the ages of 16-19 years. Women in their third and fourth decade of life may experience acne lesions on the chin or jaw line.

- Is the patient experiencing rosacea?
  - Individuals with an onset of lesions or persistence of lesions from adolescence that are in their mid-20s may be experiencing rosacea, erythema, or facial flushing located on the cheeks in the absence of comedones.

TABLE 1. Exacerbating factors in acne

Factor	Description of factor
Acne mechanica	Local irritation or friction from occlusive clothing, headbands, helmets, or other friction-producing devices
	Excessive contact between face and hands, such as resting the chin or cheek on the hand
Excoriated acne	A form of acne caused by constant picking, squeezing, or scratching at the skin, which causes the acne to look worse
Acne cosmetic	Noninflammatory comedones on the face, chin, and cheek caused by occlusion of the pilosebaceous unit by oil-based cosmetics, moisturizers, pomades, or other health and beauty products
Chloracne	An acneiform eruption caused by exposure to chlorine compounds
Occupational acne	Exposure to dirt, vaporized cooking oils, or certain industrial chemicals, such as coal tar and petroleum derivatives
Drug-induced acne	**More common**
	Anabolic steroids, bromides, corticosteroids, corticotrophin, isoniazid, lithium, phenytoin
	Less common
	Azathioprine, cyclosporine, disulfiram, phenobarbital, quinidine, tetracycline, vitamins B1, B6, B12, and D2
Stress and emotional extremes	May induce expression of neuroendocrine modulators and release of CRH, which play a role in centrally and topically induced stress of the sebaceous glands and possibly the progression of acne
High-humidity environments and prolonged sweating	Hydration-induced decrease in size of pilosebaceous duct orifice and prevention of loosening of comedones
Hormonal alterations	Increased androgen levels induced by medical conditions, pregnancy, or medications

Abbreviations used: CRH, corticotrophin-releasing hormone.

TABLE 2. Grading and classification of acne

Mild	Moderate	Severe
Few erythematous papules and occasional pustules mixed with comedones	Many erythematous papules and pustules and prominent scarring	Extensive pustules, erythematous papules, and multiple nodules in an inflamed background

- What treatments has the patient tried previously?
  - Avoid recommending medications that have been unsuccessful in the past, despite being used correctly and for the appropriate duration of time.
  - Identify patient's preference in dosage form (e.g., cream, gel, lotion) to improve adherence and outcomes of therapy.

Physical Assessment Techniques

Observe the patient's number and type of acne lesions to determine the severity of the acne. See Table 2 for a commonly used acne grading system.

QuEST: Establish that the patient is an appropriate self-care candidate

Utilize the information collected in the patient assessment with the treatment algorithm and exclusions for self-care to determine if self-care is appropriate.

Exclusions for Self-Care

Review the treatment algorithm and exclusions for self-care provided at the beginning of the chapter. This section highlights key exclusion criteria.

Medications

- Corticosteroids may sensitize follicles and cause hypertrophic changes, producing acne.

- Anabolic steroids, bromides, corticotrophin, isoniazid, lithium, and phenytoin are medications commonly associated with acne exacerbations.

- Azathioprine, cyclosporine, disulfiram, phenobarbital, quinidine, tetracycline, and vitamins B_1, B_6, B_{12}, and D_2 are medications less commonly associated with acne exacerbations.

◼ Conditions

■ Rosacea treatment often requires oral or topical antibiotics or oral isotretinoin.

■ Nonprescription medications are indicated for patients with mild, noninflammatory acne rather than moderate-to-severe acne.

◼ Special Populations

■ Patients that become pregnant or who plan to become pregnant while receiving acne treatment should be referred to their OB/GYN, as retinoids are teratogenic.

■ Pediatric patients less than 12 years of age require a differential diagnosis by a health care provider to evaluate for possible underlying medical conditions. Additionally, most medications are not approved for children under 12 years of age.

◼ ◼ QuE◼T: Suggest appropriate self-care strategies

Select the appropriate treatment option based on the patient data that was previously collected. Various treatment options are discussed along with clinical pearls and pertinent patient considerations for optimal management.

◼ Treatment Options

The mild, noninflammatory acne lesion treatment of choice is a topical retinoid or benzoyl peroxide. See Table 3 for a comparison of common nonprescription topical acne agents.

■ Retinoid
  ▪ Adapalene gel is the first retinoid available without a prescription.
  ▪ The full therapeutic effect occurs after 8-12 weeks of treatment.

TABLE 3. Comparison of common nonprescription topical acne agents

	Antibacterial	Comedolytic	Anti-inflammatory	Keratolytic
Benzoyl peroxide	√	√	—	—
Salicylic acid	—	√	—	√
Adapalene	—	√	√	√

- Adverse effects include redness, itching, dryness, scaling, and burning that is transient and likely to improve after the first month of use.

CAUTIONS FOR RETINOIDS

- Adapalene increases sun sensitivity. Recommend avoiding unnecessary sun exposure and using broad-spectrum sunscreen with an SPF 15 or higher.
- Retinoids have the potential to cause teratogenic effects; avoid use in pregnant females or those planning to become pregnant.

- Benzoyl Peroxide
  - Benzoyl peroxide prevents or eliminates the development of treatment-resistant *P. acnes.*
  - Higher concentrations have the same antibacterial effect as lower concentrations but may cause more skin irritation.
  - The full therapeutic effect occurs after 3-6 weeks of continuous therapy; continued treatment prevents new lesion formation.
  - Adverse effects include mild erythema and skin peeling that usually resolves within the first two weeks.

CAUTIONS FOR BENZOYL PEROXIDE

- Contact with clothes and hair may cause bleaching.
- Benzoyl peroxide increases sun sensitivity. Recommend avoiding unnecessary sun exposure and using broad-spectrum sunscreen with an SPF 15 or higher.
- Contact dermatitis and allergic reactions to benzoyl peroxide are rare; if either occurs, discontinue use.

Other Treatment Considerations

- Hydroxy Acids
  - Hydroxy acids are an option in patients who are unable to tolerate other topical acne medications.
  - Alpha hydroxy acids (AHAs) are a common ingredient in chemical peels.
  - The full therapeutic effect occurs after 3-6 weeks of continuous use.
  - Adverse effects include dryness and peeling.

> ### CAUTIONS FOR HYDROXY ACIDS
> - Topical salicylic acid can be systemically absorbed; chronic therapy or use over extensive areas of the body can result in salicylate toxicity.
> - Salicylic acid is chemically similar to aspirin; concurrent use with aspirin, antidiabetic agents, anticoagulants, and pyrazinamide increases the risk for toxicities.
> - Recommend avoiding unnecessary sun exposure and using broad-spectrum sunscreen with an SPF 15 or higher.
> - Contact dermatitis and allergic reactions to salicylic acid are rare; if either occurs, discontinue use.

- Sulfur
  - Sulfur alone is not highly effective; preference should be given to medications that have a combination of sulfur and resorcinol.
  - Adverse effects include noticeable odor and dry skin.

> ### CAUTIONS FOR SULFUR
> - Avoid use in patients with allergies to sulfa drugs.

- Sulfur/Resorcinol
  - Resorcinol is not effective as monotherapy; preference should be given to medications that have a combination of sulfur and resorcinol.
  - Adverse effects include dry skin and a reversible dark brown scale on some darker-skinned individuals.

> ### CAUTIONS FOR SULFUR/RESORCINOL
> - Avoid use in patients with allergies to sulfa drugs.

- *Scarring* is a physical complication of acne that can contribute to the negative psychosocial aspect of acne. A light chemical peel containing AHA may be used once acne is controlled to correct scarring and hyperpigmentation.

- Limited evidence supports the use of physical treatments such as light therapies, scrubs, brushes, heating devices, and comedone extraction strips.

- Complementary Therapy
  - Tea tree oil is known to have anti-inflammatory properties. Limited literature exists supporting the efficacy of tea tree oil in the treatment

of acne. There is some evidence to support that tea tree oil may reduce the number of acne lesions.

- Oral zinc supplements have bacteriostatic properties and have been shown to be effective against severe acne. Oral zinc supplements may be used as an alternative to tetracycline therapy in patients that can tolerate the gastrointestinal adverse effects.
- Vitamin A lacks studies to validate the claim that it works against acne. Doses that may be beneficial are limited to 300,000 units daily for women and 500,000 units daily for men.
- Nicotinamide, the active form of niacin, is believed to possess anti-inflammatory properties and helps improve skin texture and reduce sebum production. Although the pharmacology targets multiple etiologies of acne, the data supporting use is limited.

Special Populations

Pregnancy

- Pregnant women often experience acne that is potentiated by hormonal changes. Women that become pregnant while actively treating acne with a nonprescription medication should discontinue use because of the potential teratogenic effects.
- Topical benzoyl peroxide, sulfur, and hydroxyl acids are Pregnancy Risk Category C, and glycolic acid peels have not been evaluated in pregnancy; use of these medications should be done under the direction of an OB/GYN.

Breastfeeding

- Limited data exist regarding the effects of topical acne treatments on breastmilk. Nursing mothers should avoid utilizing topical acne medications in areas that come in direct contact with the nursing infant to prevent irritation.

Pediatric Patients

- Low concentration benzoyl peroxide ($\leq 2.5\%$) may be used in children as young as 9 years of age; all other concentrations should be reserved for use in children 12 years of age and older. Salicylic acid and adapalene may be used in children 12 years of age and older. The use of these agents should be done under the direction and supervision of a pediatrician or dermatologist.
- Neonates and infants may experience self-limiting acne; referral to a pediatrician to perform a differential diagnosis is recommended.

⬛ ⬛ QuES⬛: Talk with the patient

⬛ *Patient Education/Counseling*

▪ Nonpharmacologic Talking Points
- Cleanse skin with a mild, oil-free cleanser twice a day with warm water.
- Use of a skin toner removes excess dirt and oil to prevent and minimize acne flare-ups.
- Select noncomedogenic skin care products, hair care products, and cosmetics.
- Worsening of acne and scarring occur when comedones are picked at or squeezed; this should be avoided.

▪ Pharmacologic Talking Points
- General counseling points for topical acne treatments include the following:
  - Efficacy is best when contact time with skin is prolonged; this limits the effectiveness of washes and medicated cleansers.
  - Gel formulations are most effective because of their synergistic drying effect and longer contact time with skin.
  - A thin layer should be applied to the affected areas, not just to visible lesions, for prevention and treatment of acne lesions.
  - It is common for acne to worsen during the first weeks of therapy.
  - Avoid contact with mucous membranes and open wounds to limit excessive irritation.
  - To reduce the risk of sunburn, use a broad-spectrum sunscreen with a minimum SPF of 15.
  - Do not use combinations of acne medications unless directed by a dermatologist or health care provider.
- Retinoid
  - Experiencing redness, itching, dryness, and burning for the first month of therapy is common; these adverse effects are transient.
  - Discontinue use of adapalene if you are planning a pregnancy or become pregnant.
- Benzoyl Peroxide
  - To test for irritation, medications should be applied over a small area once daily for 3 days. The number of daily applications may be increased after 1-2 weeks of use, as tolerated.

- Patients may double the concentration at weekly intervals if necessary.
- Adverse effects may be managed by selecting a lower concentration or reducing the frequency of use.
- Benozyl peroxide that comes in contact with hair or fabrics may result in bleaching.

- Salicylic Acid
  - Application of topical gel formulation should be limited to the affected area.
  - Reducing the frequency of use to daily or every other day may improve excessive peeling.

- Sulfur
  - Sulfur has a distinct odor; because of its chalky consistency, a tinted product may be preferred.

- Suggest medical referral if any of the following occur:
  - Moderate-severe or inflammatory acne lesions develop.
  - There is no improvement in number, extent, or severity of acne lesions following 6 weeks of treatment with benzoyl peroxide or 3 months with adapalene.
  - Severe skin irritation or sensitivity with nonprescription medications develops.
  - There is an allergic reaction or anaphylaxis following use of any topical medication.

Clinical Pearls

- Pharmacologic and nonpharmacologic therapies should be tailored to target patient exacerbating factors and medication-specific preferences, such as formulation, number of daily applications, and tolerability of adverse effects, to maximize adherence.

- Adherence to therapy is essential for medication effectiveness and improvement in the number and severity of acne lesions; complete resolution of acne is not a realistic expectation for self-treatment.

- Women who experience acne related to hormonal fluctuations or imbalance (e.g., acne that occurs around the time of menstruation) may benefit from the use of prescription therapies, such as oral contraceptives.

■ ■ References

1. Foster KT. Acne. In: Krinsky DL, Ferreri SP, Henstreet BA, Hume AL, Newton GD, Rollins CJ, Tietze KJ, eds. *Handbook of Nonprescription Drugs: An Interactive Approach to Self-Care*. Washington, DC: American Pharmacists Association; 2017:727-742.

2. Titus S, Hodge J. Diagnosis and treatment of acne. *Am Fam Physician*. 2012;86(8):734–40.

ALLERGIC RHINITIS

Miranda Wilhelm, PharmD

For complete information about this topic, consult Chapter 11, "Colds and Allergy," written by Kelly L. Scolaro and published in the *Handbook of Nonprescription Drugs,* 19th Edition.[1]

Self-Care of Allergic Rhinitis

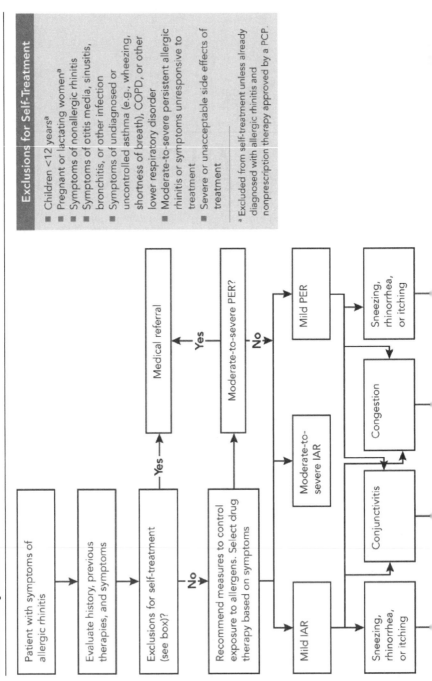

Exclusions for Self-Treatment

- Children <12 years[a]
- Pregnant or lactating women[a]
- Symptoms of nonallergic rhinitis
- Symptoms of otitis media, sinusitis, bronchitis, or other infection
- Symptoms of undiagnosed or uncontrolled asthma (e.g., wheezing, shortness of breath), COPD, or other lower respiratory disorder
- Moderate-to-severe persistent allergic rhinitis or symptoms unresponsive to treatment
- Severe or unacceptable side effects of treatment

[a] Excluded from self-treatment unless already diagnosed with allergic rhinitis and nonprescription therapy approved by a PCP.

Patient with symptoms of allergic rhinitis

Evaluate history, previous therapies, and symptoms

Exclusions for self-treatment (see box)?

Yes → Medical referral

No

Recommend measures to control exposure to allergens. Select drug therapy based on symptoms

Moderate-to-severe PER?

Yes → Medical referral

No

Mild IAR

Moderate-to-severe IAR

Mild PER

Sneezing, rhinorrhea, or itching

Conjunctivitis

Congestion

Sneezing, rhinorrhea, or itching

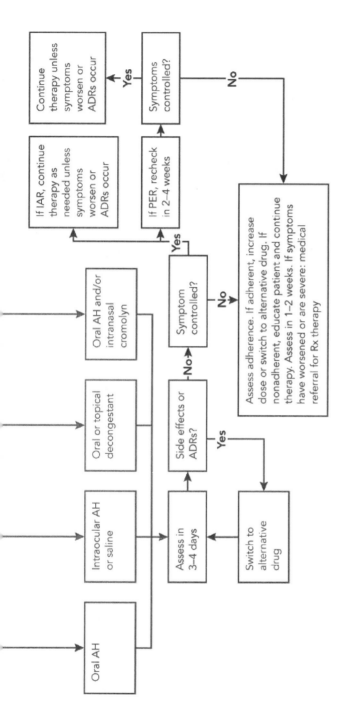

ADR = adverse drug reaction; AH = antihistamine; COPD = chronic obstructive pulmonary disease; IAR = intermittent allergic rhinitis; PCP = primary care provider; PER = persistent allergic rhinitis; Rx = prescription.

■ ■ Overview

■ Allergic rhinitis is a systemic disease with prominent nasal symptoms. It represents an immunoglobulin E (IgE) mediated response to indoor and outdoor environmental allergens.

■ Allergic rhinitis is classified by both duration and severity of symptoms. Patients are classified as having episodic, mild intermittent, moderate-to-severe intermittent, mild persistent, or moderate-to-severe persistent allergic rhinitis (see Table 1 for further descriptions).

■ Symptoms begin after the second year of life, and the disease is prevalent in children and adults 18–64 years of age. After 65 years of age, the number of cases decreases.

■ Allergic rhinitis cannot be cured. The goals of self-treatment are to reduce symptoms and improve the patient's functional status and sense of well-being.

■ ■ Pathophysiology

■ The pathogenesis of allergic rhinitis is complex, involving numerous cells and mediators, and consists of four phases:
1. Sensitization phase with initial allergen exposure and IgE production
2. Early phase within minutes of allergen exposure that consists of rapid release of preformed mast cell mediators (e.g., histamine, proteases)

TABLE 1. Classification of allergic rhinitis

Duration	Severity
Intermittent Symptoms occur ≤4 days per week OR ≤4 weeks.	**Mild** Symptoms do not impair sleep or daily activities[a]; no troublesome symptoms **Moderate-Severe** One or more of the following occurs: impairment of sleep, impairment of daily activities[a], troublesome symptoms
Persistent Symptoms occur >4 days per week AND >4 weeks.	**Mild** Symptoms do not impair sleep or daily activities[a]; no troublesome symptoms **Moderate-Severe** One or more of the following occurs: impairment of sleep, impairment of daily activities[a], troublesome symptoms
Episodic Symptoms occur if an individual is in contact with an exposure that is not normally a part of the individual's environment (e.g., a cat at a friend's house).	Can be mild, moderate, or severe, based on symptoms

[a]Daily activities include work, school, sports, and leisure.

and production of additional mediators (e.g., prostaglandins, kinins, leukotrienes, neuropeptides)

3. Cellular recruitment involving circulating leukocytes to the nasal mucosa and release of more inflammatory mediators

4. Late phase, 2–4 hours after allergen exposure, which includes mucus hypersecretion secondary to congestion

- Common outdoor aeroallergens: pollen, mold spores, pollutants, tobacco smoke.

- Common indoor aeroallergens: house-dust mites, cockroaches, mold spores, pet dander.

- Occupational aeroallergens: wool dust, latex, resins, organic dusts.

Risk Factors

- Family history of atopy (allergic disorders) in one or both parents, higher socioeconomic level, eczema, and positive reaction to allergy skin tests.

- Emerging evidence also suggests that diet may be a risk factor in children and adolescents. Children who consume 3 or more fast-food meals per week showed an increased incidence of allergic disorders.

Complications

- Acute complications include sinusitis and otitis media with effusion.

- Chronic complications include nasal polyps, sleep apnea, sinusitis, and diminished sense of smell.

QuEST: Quickly and Accurately Assess the Patient Using SCHOLAR MAC

QuEST SCHOLAR is an acronym used to assess a patient to determine self-care candidate status and to identify which treatment would be most appropriate. See Chapter 1 for a description of the QuEST SCHOLAR process.

Does the Patient Have Allergic Rhinitis?

- Paroxysmal sneezing; watery rhinorrhea; itching of the eyes, nose, palate, or combinations thereof; and conjunctivitis (red, irritated eyes with prominent conjunctival blood vessels).

- Nasal congestion is a variable finding.

- Systemic symptoms include fatigue, irritability, malaise, and cognitive impairment.

- In general, symptoms are worse upon awakening, improve during the day, and then may worsen again at night.

● Important SCHOLAR MAC Considerations

- Are symptoms more bothersome during a certain time of day? (e.g., upon waking, trouble sleeping due to symptoms)

- Are symptoms more bothersome during certain times of the year? (e.g., spring and fall)

- Are symptoms more bothersome after certain activities? (e.g., being outside, in contact with an animal)

- Is the patient experiencing nasal or sore throat symptoms or multiple symptoms?
  - Determine which symptom is the most bothersome to utilize single ingredient products as often as possible.
  - Determine if sore throat is due to drainage (postnasal drip) running down the back of the throat to utilize intranasal corticosteroids (INCS) or antihistamines.

● Physical Assessment Techniques

- Observe the patient for facial features of allergic rhinitis:
  - Allergic shiners—periorbital darkening secondary to venous congestion.
  - Dennie's lines—wrinkles beneath the lower eyelids.
  - Allergic crease—horizontal crease just above bulbar portion of the nose secondary to the "allergic salute."
  - Allergic salute—patient will rub the tip of the nose upward with the palm of the hand.
  - Allergic gape—open-mouth breathing secondary to nasal obstruction.

- Observe the patient for signs of chronic medical conditions, such as wheezing (asthma, chronic obstructive pulmonary disease [COPD]), productive cough (COPD), barrel chest (COPD), enlarged lymph nodes (general infection).

- Obtain vital signs (e.g., temperature, respiratory rate, pulse, and blood pressure).

- Palpate sinuses and neck and observe any pain or tenderness.

- Visually examine throat for redness or exudates. If bacterial pharyngitis is suspected, run rapid strep test, if available.

- Auscultate chest to detect wheezing, crackles, and rapid or irregular heartbeat.

▇ ▇ Qu▇ST: Establish that the patient is an appropriate self-care candidate

Utilize the information collected in the patient assessment with the treatment algorithm and exclusions for self-care to determine if self-care is appropriate.

▇ Exclusions to Self-Care

Review the treatment algorithm and exclusions for self-care provided at the beginning of the chapter. This section highlights key exclusion criteria.

▇ Medications

- Anticholinergics—potential treatment options can have additive effects, resulting in dryness of the eyes and mucous membranes, blurred vision, urinary hesitancy and retention, constipation, and reflex tachycardia.

- Central nervous system (CNS) depressants—potential treatment options can have additive sedation and impaired performance effects (e.g., impaired driving performance, poor work performance, incoordination, reduced motor skills, and impaired information processing). In addition, this can lead to increased risk for adverse effects and falls.

- Monoamine oxidase inhibitors (MAOI)—first-generation (sedating) antihistamines can have additive sedation, anticholinergic effects, or hypotensive reactions.

- See Table 2 for a list of common drug interactions.

▇ Conditions

- COPD, benign prostatic hyperplasia, and overactive bladder could limit medication selection due to drug-disease interactions and adverse effects.

TABLE 2. Clinically important drug–drug interactions with allergy products

Drug/Drug Class	Potential Interaction (Drug-Specific Data)	Management/Prevention
Antihistamines		
Amiodarone	Increased risk of QT interval prolongation (loratadine)	Avoid combination.
Antacids (aluminum and magnesium salts)	Decreased efficacy (fexofenadine)	Separate doses by as much time as possible.
Anticholinergics (e.g., ipratropium, tiotropium, umeclidinium)	Enhanced anticholinergic effects (dry mouth, eyes, urinary retention, sedation)	Avoid combination.
Brexpiprazole	Increased risk of brexpiprazole toxicity (diphenhydramine)	Reduce brexpiprazole dose by 25% or avoid combination.
CNS depressants (alcohol, opiates, sedatives)	Increased sedation (sedating antihistamines; cetirizine, levocetirizine)	Avoid combination.
Erythromycin; ketoconazole	Increased fexofenadine plasma concentration	Monitor therapy closely.
Metoprolol	Increased metoprolol serum concentrations and risk of hypotension (diphenhydramine)	Reduce metoprolol dose or avoid combination.
Phenytoin	Decreased phenytoin elimination (chlorpheniramine)	Monitor therapy or avoid combination.
Potassium chloride (oral)	Increased risk of ulcers	Avoid combination.
Intranasal Corticosteroids		
Protease inhibitors (e.g., ritonavir, tipranavir, telaprevir)	Increased serum concentration of steroids (budesonide, fluticasone)	Avoid combination.

■ Formulations of 12 and 24-hour sustained-release loratadine-pseudo-ephedrine combination products are contraindicated in patients with esophageal narrowing, abnormal esophageal peristalsis, or a history of difficulty swallowing tablets.

■ Special Populations

■ First-generation (sedating) antihistamines are contraindicated in newborns or premature infants.

■ Children may experience paradoxical excitation rather than sedation when taking first-generation (sedating) antihistamines.

■ First-generation (sedating) antihistamines are contraindicated in lactating women because of potential adverse effects on the infant and decreased milk production because of anticholinergic effects.

■ Frail older adults may not be candidates for first-generation (sedating) antihistamines, as they are listed on the Beer's criteria; all nonprescription medication should be considered for appropriateness and dose adjustments made as needed.

■ ■ QuE⑤T: Suggest appropriate self-care strategies

Select the appropriate treatment option based on the previously collected patient data. Various treatment options are discussed along with clinical pearls and pertinent patient considerations for optimal management.

■ Treatment Options

Nasal symptoms (e.g., itching, rhinorrhea, sneezing and congestion) treatment of choice is an INCS.

■ Intranasal Corticosteroids
- INCS are the most effective treatment for allergic rhinitis, and monotherapy is considered first-line.
- Full effect may not be seen until at least 1 week of use.
- INCS have low systemic absorption and therefore are well tolerated.
- Adverse effects associated with INCS are minor and include nasal discomfort or nosebleeds, sneezing, cough, and pharyngitis. Patients who are sensitive to INCS or use higher-than-recommended doses may experience systemic effects such as headache, dizziness, nausea, and vomiting.

> **CAUTIONS FOR INTRANASAL CORTICOSTEROIDS**
> - Long-term use has been linked to changes in vision, glaucoma, cataracts, increased risk of infection (i.e., *Candida*), and growth inhibition in children.
> - Inappropriate nasal spray technique can cause septal perforation.

■ Antihistamines
- May be used alone or in combination with INCS if symptoms are not controlled.
- Antihistamines are not effective for nasal congestion but may be used to treat pharyngitis caused by postnasal drip.
- The role of first-generation (sedating) antihistamines in treating allergic rhinitis is controversial because of the risk versus benefit analysis. Second-generation antihistamines are preferred over first-generation antihistamines in allergic rhinitis.
  - Of the second-generation antihistamines, fexofenadine and loratadine are considered nonsedating.

- Cetirizine has been shown to be more potent than fexofenadine or loratadine, but it causes sedation in approximately 10% of patients.
- Adverse effects associated with first-generation (sedating) antihistamines include CNS depression (e.g., sedation, impaired performance) and anticholinergic effects (e.g., dry eyes, mouth, nose, vagina; blurred vision; urinary hesitancy and retention; constipation; and reflex tachycardia) but are rarely seen with second-generation (nonsedating) agents.

CAUTIONS FOR ANTIHISTAMINES

- First-generation (sedating) antihistamines are listed as Potentially Inappropriate Medications for Older Adults in the 2015 American Geriatrics Society Beers Criteria.[2] The AGS recommends avoiding use in older adults.
- Narrow-angle glaucoma, acute asthma exacerbation, stenosing peptic ulcer, symptomatic prostatic hypertrophy, bladder neck and pyloroduodenal obstruction are contraindications to use of first-generation (sedating) antihistamines.
- First-generation (sedating) antihistamines are photosensitizing drugs and require use of sunscreen or protective clothing.
- Fexofenadine should not be taken with any fruit juices (e.g., grapefruit, apple, or orange), as juice reduces fexofenadine absorption. Separation by at least 2 hours will avoid this interaction.
- While tolerance to antihistamines is not likely, other factors may contribute, including patient nonadherence, increased antigen exposure, worsening of disease, limited effectiveness of antihistamines in severe disease, or the development of similar symptoms from unrelated disease. Suggest switching to a different class of antihistamine if the patient has a less-than-optimal response.

Intranasal Mast Cell Stabilizer

- Cromolyn sodium (intranasal cromolyn) is the nonprescription mast cell stabilizer spray for allergic rhinitis.
- Treatment is more effective if started before symptoms begin. It may take 3–7 days for initial clinical improvement to become apparent and 2–4 weeks of continued therapy to achieve maximal therapeutic benefit.
- Intranasal mast cell stabilizers have minimal systemic absorption with no systemic activity and are well tolerated.

- Adverse effects associated with mast cell stabilizers include nasal discomfort (e.g., sneezing, nasal stinging and burning).

CAUTIONS FOR INTRANASAL MAST CELL STABILIZER

- No drug interactions have been reported with intranasal cromolyn.

Nasal congestion not controlled by INCS may be treated with systemic or short-term (≤5 days) use of topical decongestants.

- Decongestants
  - Decongestants have little effect on other symptoms of allergic rhinitis.
  - Combination products with second-generation (nonsedating) antihistamines offer convenience but should be used with caution because of the increased risk of adverse effects.

CAUTIONS FOR DECONGESTANTS

- Patients with hypertension should use systemic decongestants only with medical advice.
- Decongestants are contraindicated in patients receiving concomitant MAOIs and for 2 weeks after discontinuation.
- Persons taking selective serotonin reuptake inhibitor (SSRI) or serotonin and norepinephrine reuptake inhibitor (SNRI) antidepressants should use decongestants with caution, as these medications may increase heart rate.

Ocular symptoms (such as itching, redness, and watery discharge) may be treated with an INCS (fluticasone furoate and propionate have additional FDA approval for ophthalmic symptoms).

- Complementary Therapy
  - Parthenolide, feverfew's biologically active component, may have anti-inflammatory properties, but its safety and efficacy in allergic rhinitis are unproven.
  - Some homeopathic products intended for the treatment of allergic rhinitis actually contain known allergens (e.g., bioAllers Animal Hair and Dander Allergy Relief Liquid contains cat, cattle, dog, horse, and sheep wool extracts). Using these products to induce long-term resistance by repeated exposure to controlled amounts of allergen has not been proven to be safe or effective.

Special Populations

Pregnancy

- Pregnancy is a common cause of nonallergic rhinitis; thus, pregnant women should be referred for differential diagnosis.
- If allergic rhinitis is confirmed and nonprescription therapy is approved by an OB/GYN, intranasal cromolyn is considered compatible with pregnancy and is a first-line option.
- Diphenhydramine and chlorpheniramine are considered compatible with pregnancy.
- Levocetirizine, loratadine, and cetirizine are considered to carry a low risk of adverse fetal effects. Fexofenadine is associated with moderate risk and should not be recommended.
- INCS are considered compatible with pregnancy because of their minimal systemic absorption. However, systemic use of budesonide and triamcinolone has been linked to cleft lip and palate and low birth weight.

Breastfeeding

- Lactating women approved for self-treatment by an OB/GYN can use intranasal cromolyn. With limited systemic absorption, it is a good choice, and adverse effects in nursing infants have not been reported.
- INCS are thought to be excreted in breast milk. Reports of INCS causing harm in nursing infants are lacking, however, and they are considered "probably compatible."
- Antihistamines are contraindicated during lactation because of their ability to pass into breast milk. Short-acting chlorpheniramine, fexofenadine, or loratadine are the best options if an oral antihistamine is needed. If an oral antihistamine is used during lactation, the mother should avoid long-acting and high-dose antihistamines and should take the dose at bedtime after the last feeding of the day.

Pediatric Patients

- Because of concerns regarding undiagnosed asthma, children less than 12 years of age should be referred to a pediatrician for differential diagnosis.
- Intranasal cromolyn, fluticasone furoate, and triamcinolone acetonide are safe for children 2 years of age and older.
- Intranasal fluticasone propionate is safe for children 4 years of age and older.
- Intranasal budesonide is safe for children 6 years of age and older.

- Intranasal products may be difficult for children to self-administer. In addition, INCS have been linked to growth inhibition in children; FDA-mandated labeling for nonprescription products encourages parents to speak to a health care provider if they plan to use these products in children for 2 months or longer per year.
- Loratadine is the nonprescription antihistamine of choice, followed by fexofenadine, levocetirizine, and cetirizine.

- Geriatric Patients
    - Older adults are more likely than other age groups to experience adverse effects with first-generation (sedating) antihistamines. As these drugs are included in the Beers Criteria, they should be avoided. Those adverse effects contribute to a higher risk of falling in this population.
    - Loratadine and intranasal cromolyn are drugs of choice in older adults. Dosage of fexofenadine and levocetirizine should be adjusted in patients with renal impairment. Loratadine and cetirizine dosage should be adjusted in patients with renal or hepatic impairment, or both.

■ ● QuESⓣ: Talk with the patient

● Patient Education/Counseling

- Nonpharmacologic Points
    - Allergen avoidance is the primary nonpharmacologic measure for allergic rhinitis. Avoidance strategies depend on the specific allergen (see Table 3 for detailed approaches).
    - Nasal wetting agents or nasal irrigation with warm saline delivered using a syringe or neti pot may relieve nasal irritation and dryness and aid in the removal of dried, encrusted, or thick mucus from the nose. Only distilled, sterile, or boiled tap water should be used to prepare nasal irrigation solutions because of the risk of rare but serious infections.

- Pharmacologic Points
    - Agents with different mechanisms of action or delivery systems may be added if single-drug therapy does not provide adequate relief, or if symptoms are already moderately severe, particularly intense, or long-lasting.

TABLE 3. Allergen avoidance strategies

General
- Consider weekly vacuuming of carpets, drapes, and upholstery with a high-efficiency particulate air (HEPA) filter-equipped vacuum cleaner.
- Change filters in ventilation systems regularly.

House Dust Mites (*Dermatophagoides* spp.)
- Reduce household humidity to <40%.
- Apply acaricides.
- Reduce mite-harboring dust by removing carpets, upholstered furniture, stuffed animals, and bookshelves from the patient's bedroom and other rooms, if possible.
- Reduce mite populations in bedding by encasing the mattress, box springs, and pillows with mite-impermeable materials. Bedding that cannot be encased should be washed at least weekly in hot (131°F [55°C]) water. Bedding that cannot be encased or laundered should be discarded.

Mold Spores
- Avoid outdoor activities that disturb decaying plant material.
- Reduce household humidity.
- Remove houseplants.
- Vent food preparation areas and bathrooms.
- Repair damp basements or crawl spaces.
- Apply fungicide frequently to obviously moldy areas.

Cat-Derived Allergens
- Although unproven, weekly cat baths may reduce the allergen load.

Cockroaches
- Keep areas clean.
- Store food tightly sealed.
- Treat infested areas with baits or pesticides.

Pollutants
- Avoid outdoor activities when the AQI (air quality index—a measure of five major air pollutants per 24 hours) is high.

Pollen
- Anticipate peak times for bothersome pollen allergens: trees pollinate in spring, grasses in early summer, and ragweed from mid-August to the first fall frost.
- Avoid outdoor activities when pollen counts are very high (generally early in the morning and in the evening).
- Close house and car windows to reduce pollen exposure.

- Intranasal Corticosteroids
  - Patient should be instructed to prime the spray before the first use and when it has not been used for a week or more.
  - Patients should be instructed to shake the bottle gently before use to ensure suspension is mixed and uniform.
  - INCS may irritate the nose, or the bottle tip can injure the nose if used forcefully.

- INCS are effective for itchy eyes and nose, sneezing, runny nose, and congestion.
- While the medication starts working right away, it may take 1 week for maximal effect.
- INCS are more effective when used regularly rather than episodically.
- Antihistamines
  - Antihistamines are effective for itching, sneezing, and runny nose but have little effect on nasal congestion.
  - First-generation (sedating) antihistamines can cause drowsiness, impaired mental alertness, and anticholinergic effects; therefore, the potential benefits of the medication must be weighed against the potential risks.
- Intranasal Mast Cell Stabilizer
  - While the medication starts working right away, it may take 1–2 weeks for maximal effect.

- Suggest medical referral if any of the following occur:
  - Symptoms that worsen while taking nonprescription medications or do not decrease after 2–4 weeks of treatment.
  - Patients who do not respond to nonprescription therapy should be referred back to their primary care provider for prescription medications, such as intranasal antihistamines, systemic corticosteroids, leukotriene inhibitors, anticholinergics, or immunotherapy
  - Symptoms of a secondary bacterial infection (e.g., thick nasal or respiratory secretions that are not clear, oral temperature higher than 101.5°F [38.6°C], shortness of breath, chest congestion, wheezing, significant ear pain, rash).

Clinical Pearls

- Patients with intermittent allergic rhinitis should start treatment with INCS, antihistamines, intranasal cromolyn, or combinations thereof at least 1 week before symptoms typically appear or as soon as possible before known allergen exposure. Therapy should continue as long as the allergen is present.

- Patients with situational allergic rhinitis (e.g., occasional animal exposure) should take a second-generation (nonsedating) antihistamine 3 hours before known allergen exposure for symptom control. Daily use is not necessary.

■ ■ References

5. Scolaro K. Colds and Allergy. In: Krinsky DL, Ferreri SP, Hemstreet BA, Hume AL, Newton GD, Rollins CJ, Tietze KJ, eds. *Handbook of Nonprescription Drugs: An Interactive Approach to Self-Care.* Washington, DC: American Pharmacists Association; 2017:189–216.

6. American Geriatrics Society 2015 Beers Criteria Update Expert Panel. American Geriatrics Society 2015 Updated Beers Criteria for Potentially Inappropriate Medication Use in Older Adults. *J Am Geriatr Soc.* 2015 Nov;63(11):2227–2246

BURNS AND SUNBURN

Erin N. Adams, PharmD, BCACP

For complete information about this topic, consult Chapter 41, "Minor Burns, Sunburns and Wounds," written by Daphne B. Bernard and published in the *Handbook of Nonprescription Drugs*, 19th Edition.[1]

Self-Care of Burns and Sunburn

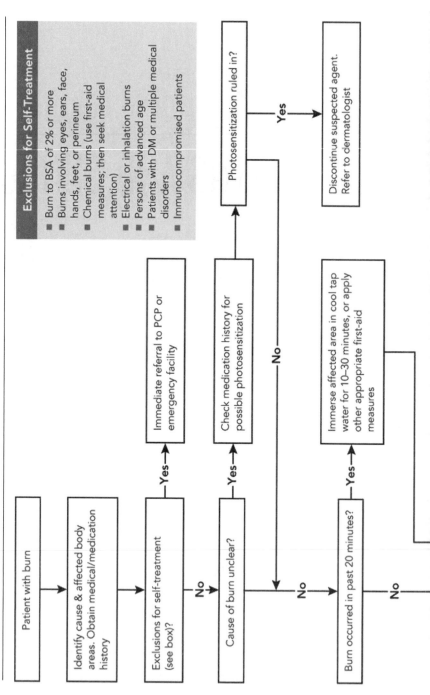

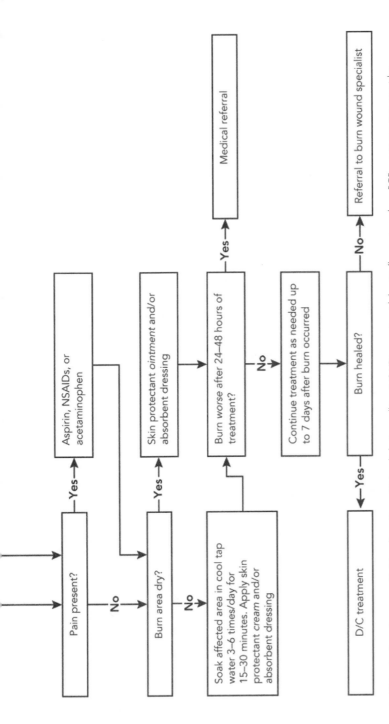

BSA = body surface area; D/C = discontinue; DM = diabetes mellitus; NSAID = nonsteroidal anti-inflammatory drug; PCP = primary care provider.

■ ● Overview

- Burns may be caused by thermal, electrical, chemical, or ultraviolet radiation (UVR) exposure.

- Healthy skin is well adapted to heal minor burns over time.

- The use of proper dressing and appropriate care will facilitate healing, minimize scar formation, and prevent secondary bacterial skin infections.

- The goals of self-treatment are to relieve symptoms, promote healing by protecting the burn from infection and further trauma, and minimize scarring.

■ ● Pathophysiology

- Minor burns and sunburns tend to heal within 1 month in healthy adults with proper care.

- Sunburns are caused by too much exposure to UVR, including ultraviolet A (UVA) and ultraviolet B (UVB) light produced from natural sunlight and by commercial tanning beds and sunlamps.[2]
  - UVA radiation penetrates the skin deeply and is responsible for tanning and photoaging of the skin.
  - UVB plays a role in the development of skin cancers and drug-induced photoallergies and photosensitivity as well as the erythema associated with sunburn.

- The most important systemic factors that can affect the healing process are poor vascularization, bacterial contamination, inadequate nutrition, coexisting medical conditions, and medications.

● *Preventative Measures*

- To prevent UVA and UVB exposure, patients should be advised to stay indoors or use physical sun protection, including wearing a hat, long pants, a long-sleeved shirt, or special sun protective clothing embedded with agents that absorb UVR. For patients 6 months of age and older, broad spectrum sunscreen with an SPF of 15 or more should be recommended. In an average adult wearing a bathing suit, 9 portions of sunscreen, each about ½ teaspoonful, should be applied to the body.
  - Patients with a sun-induced skin disorder or taking a photosensitizing agent should use SPF 30+.

- Patients with an allergic reaction to sun protectant should use sunscreen with avobenzone of SPF 15+.[2]

▪ ▪ QuEST: Quickly and Accurate Assess the Patient Using SCHOLAR MAC

QuEST SCHOLAR is an acronym used to assess a patient to determine self-care candidate status and to identify which treatment would be most appropriate. See Chapter 1 for a description of the QuEST SCHOLAR process.

▪ Does the Patient Have a Minor Burn or Sunburn?

- Minor sunburn and superficial burns involve only the epidermis, with no loss of any skin layers, and consist primarily of reddened, nonblanching, unbroken, nonblistering skin.

- Painful erythema and slight dermal edema may occur approximately 4 hours after exposure, peaking between 12–24 hours after exposure.

- In addition to the symptoms from a minor burn, blistering or partial-thickness skin loss and peeling that involves all the epidermis and part of the dermis may occur with severe burns and sunburns over a period of several days.

- Bacterial infections may occur because of the loss of the outer skin barrier.

- Systemic symptoms such as vomiting, low-grade fever, chills, weakness, and shock may be seen in patients in whom a large portion of the skin surface has been affected.

- See Table 1 for the classification and characteristics of skin burns.

▪ Important SCHOLAR MAC Considerations

- Is the burn dry or wet in appearance?
  - Determining this characteristic will help determine if a cream or ointment should be applied as treatment.

- When did the burn occur?
  - The initial appearance of the injury may be underestimated if the burn recently occurred, since the inflammatory response evolves over the first 24–48 hours.
  - Burns that fail to heal within 2–3 weeks after the initial injury are an exclusion to self-treatment.

TABLE 1. Classification and characteristics of burns

Variable	Type of Burn			
	Superficial	**Superficial Partial-Thickness**	**Deep Partial-Thickness**	**Full-Thickness**
Depth of injury	Epidermis only	Epidermis and part of dermis	Epidermis and majority of dermis	Epidermis and dermis; may involve subcutaneous tissue
Common causes	■ Brief exposure to low heat ■ Sunburn	■ Splash or spill of hot liquid ■ Brief contact with hot object ■ Flash ignition ■ Severe sunburn	■ Splash or spill of hot liquid ■ Brief contact with hot object ■ Flash ignition ■ Chemical contact ■ Exposure to flame	■ Immersion in hot liquid ■ Exposure to flame ■ Exposure to electricity ■ Chemical contact
Appearance	■ Redness, slight edema ■ Typically without blister formation	■ Redness, blistering ■ Skin may blanch with pressure (lighten in color when pressed with a finger)	■ Patchy white to red ■ Large blisters may be present	■ Dry, leathery area that is painless and insensate
Pain	Yes	Yes	Yes, sensitivity to temperature and air	No
Healing	Usually within 3–6 days	Generally within 2–3 weeks with minimal or no scarring	Longer timer period of up to 6 weeks with scarring possible	Occurs slowly over months with scarring typical
Amenable to self-treatment	Yes (thermal burns and sunburn)	Some (small thermal burns and sunburn only)	No (requires emergency department evaluation)	No (requires hospitalization)

- Where is the burn?
  - Determining how much of the body has a burn will help determine if a patient can be treated with self-care.

Physical Assessment Techniques

- Inspect the type, depth, extent, and location of the patient's burn or sunburn.

- Inspect for signs of erythema, blistering, or dermal edema or if it is wet or dry in appearance.

- Inspect for signs of infection, including whether drainage of yellow or greenish fluid is present.

QuEST: Establish that the patient is an appropriate self-care candidate

Utilize the information collected in the patient assessment with the treatment algorithm and exclusions for self-care to determine if self-care is appropriate.

Exclusions to Self-Care

Review the treatment algorithm and exclusions for self-care provided at the beginning of the chapter. This section highlights key exclusion criteria.

Medications

- Glucocorticoids – may impact tissue repair through anti-inflammatory effects.

- Chemotherapy – can impact the healing process through a variety of pathways.

Conditions

- Diabetes, severe anemia, hypotension, peripheral vascular disease, and congestive heart failure may have delayed healing and reduced resistance to infection.

Special Populations

- The Rule of Nines, which is used to estimate the body surface area (BSA) affected by a burn, is inaccurate in children and patients with small BSAs.

■ ■ QuE⑤T: Suggest appropriate self-care strategies

Select the appropriate treatment option based on the previously collected patient data. Various treatment options are discussed along with clinical pearls and pertinent patient considerations for optimal management.

■ Treatment Options

Pain and inflammation treatment of choice is early application of nonpharmacologic therapy and short-term administration of systemic analgesics.

■ Systemic Analgesics
- Analgesics, preferably with anti-inflammatory activity such as non-steroidal anti-inflammatory drugs (NSAIDs; e.g., aspirin, naproxen, or ibuprofen), are recommended to help reduce inflammation, especially in the first 24 hours after overexposure to UVR.
- For patients who cannot take NSAIDs, acetaminophen can provide pain relief.
- Adverse effects associated with oral NSAIDs include heartburn, dyspepsia, anorexia, epigastric pain, bleeding and bruising, and increased blood pressure.
- Adverse effects associated with acetaminophen include nausea, hepatotoxicity, and skin rash (rare). It is well-tolerated when recommended doses are not exceeded.

CAUTIONS FOR SYSTEMIC ANALGESICS

- Chronic use of NSAIDs can cause nephropathy, bleeding, increased cardiovascular events (e.g., myocardial infarction, stroke, heart failure), and gastrointestinal ulcerations, among other risks.
- Gastrointestinal risks are greatest in patients 60 years of age or older, patients with a history of peptic ulcer disease, patients who consume 3 or more alcoholic beverages/day, and patients who take higher doses or undergo a longer duration of treatment, or both.
- Risks may outweigh the benefits in patients 75 years and older; topical NSAIDs should be considered.
- Hepatoxicity can occur when doses exceed 4 grams/day, particularly with chronic use.
- More conservative dosing (≤2 grams/day) should be considered in the following patients: those with liver disease, taking concurrent hepatoxic drug(s), and consuming 3 or more alcoholic beverages/day.

- Potential hidden sources of acetaminophen should be identified and discouraged (e.g., Tylenol PM).
- Manufacturer labeling has decreased the daily recommended dose for all patients to 3,000–3,250 mg/day to decrease the risk of accidental overdose.

Skin dryness treatment of choice is application of a skin protectant ointment.

- Skin Protectant Ointment
    - Apply as needed to burn or sunburned skin that is dry.
    - Skin protectants are well tolerated and not associated with adverse effects.

CAUTIONS FOR SKIN PROTECTANT

- Skin protectants are recommended for use on clean, dry burns, as opposed to burns that are unclean or have excessive moisture, to prevent impaired wound healing or infection. Application of an ointment to wet burns will not allow the ointment to adhere to the skin.
- Application of an ointment too soon after a burn may trap the heat under the skin, increasing the severity of the burn.[3]

Skin wetness treatment of choice is application of a skin protectant cream.

- Skin Protectant Cream
    - Apply as needed to a burn or sunburned skin that is wet.
    - Skin protectant creams are well tolerated and not associated with adverse effects.

Preventing secondary skin infections treatment of choice is application of topical first aid antibiotics.

- Topical First Aid Antibiotics
    - Dosage form selection should be done based on the appearance of the skin (e.g., for dry skin, use an ointment; for wet skin, use a cream).
    - Adverse effects are not common, but allergic contact dermatitis (e.g., erythema, infiltration of macrophages, papules, edematous, or vesicular reaction) may occur, especially with neomycin.

CAUTIONS FOR TOPICAL ANTIBIOTICS

- Topical antibiotics are for the prevention of infections, not treatment. Burns that are infected should be referred to a primary care provider.
- Special caution should be taken when applying topical antibiotic preparations to large areas of denuded skin because the potential for systemic toxicity can increase.
- Prolonged use of these agents may result in the development of resistant bacteria and secondary fungal infection.

Other Treatment Considerations

- *Pain* associated with burns and sunburn can also be treated with topical anesthetics.
    - Relief is short-lived, lasting only 15–45 minutes. Cannot provide continuous pain relief.
    - Higher concentrations of topical anesthetics are appropriate for skin injuries in which the skin is intact. Lower concentrations are preferred when the skin surface is not intact because drug absorption is enhanced.

CAUTIONS FOR TOPICAL ANESTHETICS

- Increasing the number of applications increases the risk of hypersensitivity and systemic toxicity.
- Benzocaine has a higher incidence of hypersensitivity reactions.

Complementary Therapy

- Vitamin C has many roles in tissue repair, while a deficiency of Vitamin C may lead to an impaired immune response and increased susceptibility to infection.
- Vitamin E has anti-inflammatory properties and has been suggested to have a role in decreasing excess scar formation.
- Aloe vera gel is often found in skin products and contains vitamins A, B, C, and E. Studies using aloe vera have demonstrated variable results.
- *Calendula officinalis* is thought to promote healing by its reported anti-inflammatory and antibacterial properties. Limited studies are available.

- The use of honey may deliver a moist healing environment and has antibacterial, anti-inflammatory, and antifungal properties. One prospective randomized trial of honey versus silver sulfadiazine (SSD) for superficial burns demonstrated that honey dressings showed greater efficacy over SSD cream for treating superficial and partial-thickness burns. However, honey dressings are not advocated by burn centers.

Special Populations

- Pregnancy
  - NSAID use for inflammation or analgesia should be avoided during pregnancy.

- Geriatric Patients
  - Older adults may experience a temporary delay in healing, but quality of healing is not impacted.

QuEST: Talk with the patient

Patient Education/Counseling

- Nonpharmacologic Talking Points
  - Remove exposure to the offending agent causing the burn, stop bleeding and weeping from exudates, decrease infection risk, and protect the area from further trauma.
  - If a burn occurred in the past 20 minutes, cool the burn by immersing the area in cool tap water for 10–30 minutes.
  - Avoid the direct application of ice or ice-cold water to the burn, because this may cause numbness and intense vasoconstriction, resulting in further tissue damage.
  - In a chemical burn, prior to seeking medical attention, the area should be irrigated with copious amounts of water.
    - Clothing that has been exposed to chemicals, if not adherent to the skin, should be removed to prevent continued burns to the area. Any clothing that has to be pulled over the head should be cut off.[4]
  - If a burn involves the eye, irrigation of the eye should allow the flow of the water to go from the nasal side of the eye to the outside corner to prevent washing the contaminant into the other eye. The area poison control center should be contacted immediately at 800-222-1222, and there should be a medical referral for treatment.

- Do not break blisters or pull at burned skin because viable skin may be removed in the process, thereby delaying healing.
- It is ideal to use wound dressing to create a moist wound environment; however, if it is too wet, it may result in maceration of the tissue.
  - Gauze may be used for minor burns that are draining but must be held in place by a second agent and changed often to prevent drying of the area. Change the dressing only when it is dirty or not intact.
  - Antimicrobial dressings contain products like silver and iodine and are often used in the management of burns that are infected.
  - Specialty dressings are available that absorb excess moisture (e.g., foams, alginates), maintain moisture (e.g., hydrocolloid and transparent film dressings), or provide moisture where it is lacking (e.g., hydrogels).
- Burned skin is more susceptible to a sunburn for several weeks after initial injury. Avoiding sun exposure and using sunscreen agents during this period are recommended.

- Pharmacologic Talking Points
  - Product Application
    - To prevent contamination of any topical product, the patient should be instructed to apply the product to a clean or gloved hand or gauze and then to the burn. Do not apply products directly from the container onto the burn or sunburn.
    - Do not apply products containing camphor, menthol, or ichthammol to the burn.
    - Ointments help keep the intact skin from drying.
    - Creams allow some fluid to pass through the film and are best for broken skin.
    - Gels may dry into a smooth film coating quickly.
    - Lotions spread easily and are easier to apply when the burn area is large.
    - Aerosol and pump sprays preclude the need to physically touch the injured area, thereby decreasing the pain associated with application. However, sprays may be drying to the area and should be applied approximately 6 inches from the burn, spraying for 1–3 seconds.
  - Skin Protectants
    - Used to hold in moisture to the burn or sunburn.
    - Apply as needed.

- Topical Anesthetics
    - Wear gloves or wash hands after application to avoid anesthetic reaction to areas other than intended location.
    - Apply to the affected area no more than 3–4 times daily. Relief is short-lived, lasting only 15–45 minutes. Increasing the number of applications increases the risk of a hypersensitivity reaction and the chance for systemic toxicity.
- Topical Antibiotics
    - First-aid antibiotics are used to prevent infections. They are not indicated for the treatment of burns that are already infected.
    - Topical antibiotic preparations should be applied to the burn after cooling the area and before applying a sterile dressing.
    - Apply to the affected area no more than 3 times daily.

- Suggest medical referral if any of the following occur:
    - Report immediately to a primary care provider if the injury extends beyond the boundaries of the original burn and includes inflammation, pain, or swelling.
    - If the burn worsens or is not healed significantly after 7 days.
        - In more severe burns, medical referral is warranted again if it takes longer than 6 weeks to heal.
    - If a skin rash, weight gain, swelling, or fecal blood occurs while taking pain relievers.

Clinical Pearls

- The severity of the burn should be immediately assessed by determining the depth of the injury and the percentage of BSA involved. An easy way to estimate the percentage of burned BSA in adults is to use the back of the hand as 1% of BSA.

- Reassess burns 24–48 hours after the initial burn as the inflammatory response evolves over the first 2 days.

References

1. Bernard D. Minor Burns, Sunburn, and Wounds. In: Krinsky DL, Ferreri SP, Henstreet BA, Hume AL, Newton GD, Rollins CJ, Tietze KJ, eds. *Handbook of Nonprescription Drugs: An Interactive Approach to Self-Care.* Washington, DC: American Pharmacists Association; 2017:771–791.

2. Crosby KM, O'Neal KS. Prevention of Sun-Induced Skin Disorders. In: Krinsky DL, Ferreri SP, Henstreet BA, Hume AL, Newton GD, Rollins CJ, Tietze KJ, eds. *Handbook of Nonprescription Drugs: An Interactive Approach to Self-Care*. Washington, DC: American Pharmacists Association; 2017:743–756.

3. American Academy of Dermatology Association. Treating Sunburn. https://www.aad.org/public/kids/skin/skin-cancer/treating-sunburn. Accessed June 8, 2018.

4. Centers for Disease Control and Prevention. Chemical Agents: Facts About Personal Cleaning and Disposal of Contaminated Clothing. 2014. https://emergency.cdc.gov/planning/personalcleaningfacts.asp. Accessed September 17, 2017.

CANKER SORE (RECURRENT APHTHOUS STOMATITIS)

Karen Steinmetz Pater, PharmD, CDE, BCACP

For complete information about this topic, consult Chapter 32, "Orofacial Pain and Discomfort," written by Nicole Paolini Albanese and Mark Donaldson and published in the *Handbook of Nonprescription Drugs*, 19th edition.[1]

Self-Care of Recurrent Aphthous Stomatitis

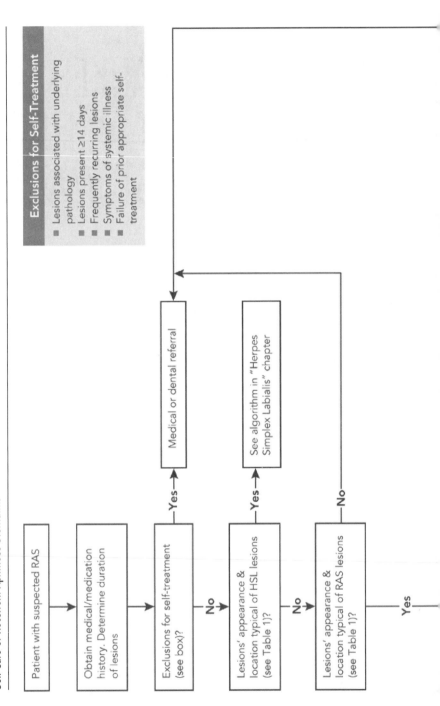

Exclusions for Self-Treatment

- Lesions associated with underlying pathology
- Lesions present ≥14 days
- Frequently recurring lesions
- Symptoms of systemic illness
- Failure of prior appropriate self-treatment

Patient with suspected RAS

↓

Obtain medical/medication history. Determine duration of lesions

↓

Exclusions for self-treatment (see box)?

— Yes → Medical or dental referral

No ↓

Lesions' appearance & location typical of HSL lesions (see Table 1)?

— Yes → See algorithm in "Herpes Simplex Labialis" chapter

No ↓

Lesions' appearance & location typical of RAS lesions (see Table 1)?

No →

Yes ↓

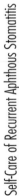

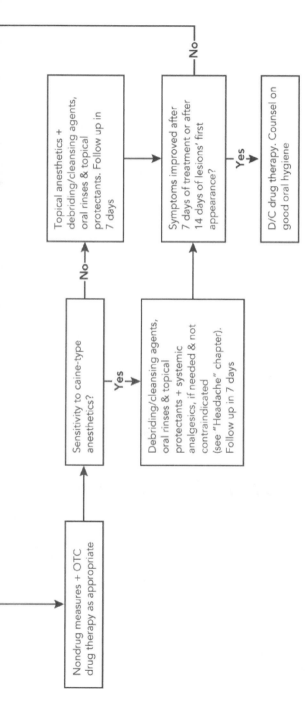

D/C = discontinue; HSL = herpes simplex labialis; OTC = over-the-counter; RAS = recurrent aphthous stomatitis.

■ ■ Overview

- Recurrent aphthous stomatitis (RAS), also known as canker sores, manifests as epithelial ulceration on nonkeratinized mucosal surfaces of movable mouth parts, such as the tongue, floor of the mouth, soft palate, or inside lining of the lips and cheeks.

- The lesions are not contagious, and they cannot be cured.

- The goals of self-treatment are to relieve pain, discomfort, and irritation so that the lesions can heal and the patient can eat, drink, and perform routine oral hygiene.

■ ■ Pathophysiology

- The cause of RAS is mostly unknown, but precipitating factors have been proposed.
  - Precipitating factors may be local, systemic, genetic, allergic, or nutritional.

- Local trauma (e.g., smoking, chemical irritation, biting the inside of cheek or lips, or injury caused by tooth brushing or braces) is the leading cause of RAS.

- The lesions will heal spontaneously if left untreated in 10–14 days.

■ ■ QuEST: Quickly and Accurate Assess the Patient Using SCHOLAR MAC

QuEST SCHOLAR is an acronym used to assess a patient to determine self-care candidate status and to identify which treatment would be most appropriate. See Chapter 1 for a description of the QuEST SCHOLAR process.

■ Does the Patient Have RAS?

- Presence of round or oval lesions on the mucosal surfaces of the mouth, such as the tongue, soft palate, floor of the mouth, or inside lining of the lips and cheeks.

- The lesions are either flat or have a depressed, crater-like appearance.

- The lesions are gray to grayish yellow in color and are surrounded by erythematous inflamed tissue.

- The lesions can be painful, with pain intensifying upon eating or drinking.

⬤ *Important SCHOLAR MAC Considerations*

- Does the patient describe a pricking or burning sensation at the site that may have occurred up to 48 hours prior to appearance of the lesion?
  - Patients may experience a prodrome that occurs 2–48 hours prior to appearance of the lesion.

- Does the patient have a fever?
  - If fever is found, this may be indicative of a secondary bacterial infection, and patients should be referred to a healthcare provider.

- Does the patient have severe pain associated with the lesions? Are the lesions found at the junction of oral mucosa and skin of lip?
  - RAS should not be confused with cold sores or fever blisters caused by Herpes Simplex Labialis (HSL). See Table 1 for differentiation of RAS and HSL.

TABLE 1. Differentiation of RAS and HSL

| Feature | RAS (Canker Sores) | | | HSL (Cold Sores) |
	Minor	Major	Herpetiform	
Clinical manifestation	Oval, flat ulcer; erythematous tissue around ulcer	Oval, ragged, gray or yellow ulcers; crateriform	Small, oval ulcers in crops; similar to minor RAS	Red, fluid-filled vesicles; lesions may coalesce; crusted when mature
Location	All areas except gingiva, hard palate, vermilion border (at junction of oral mucosa and external skin)	Any intraoral area, but predilection for lips, soft palate, and throat	Any intraoral area	Junction of oral mucosa and skin of lip and nose
Incidence	13%–26%	1.5%–3%	0.5%–1%	20%–30%
Incidence among RAS sufferers	80%	10%	5%–10%	n/a
Number of lesions	1–5	Several (1–10)	10–100 (in crops)	Several
Size of lesion	<0.5 cm	>0.5 cm	<0.5 cm	1–3 mm
Duration	10–14 days	≥6 weeks	7–10 days	10–14 days
Pain	None-moderate	None-moderate	Moderate-severe	None-moderate
Scarring	None	Common	None	Rare
Comments	Immunologic defect	Immunologic defect	Immunologic defect	Induced by HSV-1

Abbreviations used: HSV-1, herpes simplex virus type 1; n/a, not applicable.

■ Physical Assessment Techniques

■ Observe the location of lesions, number of lesions present, and size of lesions.

■ ■ Qu**E**ST: Establish that the patient is an appropriate self-care candidate

Utilize the information collected in the patient assessment with the treatment algorithm and exclusions for self-care to determine if self-care is appropriate.

■ Exclusions to Self-Care

Review the treatment algorithm and exclusions for self-care provided at the beginning of the chapter. This section highlights key exclusion criteria.

■ Conditions

■ Behcet's disease, systemic lupus erythematosus, neutrophil dysfunction, inflammatory bowel disease, and HIV/AIDS are systemic conditions known to be associated with RAS.

■ Gluten-sensitive enteropathy and deficiencies of iron and B vitamins are nutritional conditions associated with RAS.

■ ■ Qu**ES**T: Suggest appropriate self-care strategies

Select the appropriate treatment option based on the previously collected patient data. Various treatment options are discussed along with clinical pearls and pertinent patient considerations for optimal management.

■ Treatment Options

Pain, discomfort, and irritation associated with RAS may be treated with oral debriding and wound-cleansing agents, topical oral anesthetics, topical oral protectants, oral rinses, and systemic analgesics.

■ Oral Debriding and Wound-Cleansing Agents
   ■ Active ingredients include hydrogen peroxide and carbamide peroxide.

- These products should be used no longer than 7 days.
- Hydrogen peroxide 3% requires dilution prior to use.
- Adverse effects are minimal but could include soft tissue irritation.

> ### CAUTIONS FOR ORAL DEBRIDING AND WOUND-CLEANSING AGENTS
> - Prolonged rinsing with these products can lead to transient tooth sensitivity from decalcification of enamel, cellular changes, and overgrowth of undesirable organisms that could lead to the development of a black hairy tongue.

- **Topical Oral Anesthetics**
  - Active ingredients include benzocaine, benzyl alcohol, butacaine sulfate, dyclonine, hexylresorcinol, and salicylic alcohol in varying concentrations.
  - These products are often applied with an applicator that is included in the packaging.
  - Adverse effects are minimal but may include a bad taste in the mouth.

> ### CAUTIONS FOR TOPICAL ORAL ANESTHETICS
> - Patients with known hypersensitivity to benzocaine or other local anesthetics should avoid use.
> - Rare and sometimes fatal cases of methemoglobinemia have been reported with the use of topical or oromucosal benzocaine products.
> - Avoid concurrent use of benzocaine products with other drugs that can cause methemoglobin formation, such as prilocaine, nitrates, or sulfonamides.
> - Avoid using these products on open lesions due to the potential for systemic toxicity.

- **Topical Oral Protectants**
  - Active ingredients of these products are mostly inert but may include menthol and glycyrrhiza (licorice) extract.
  - These products create a barrier by using a paste, adhering film, or dissolvable patch to cover the lesion.
  - Adverse effects are minimal but may include a bad taste in the mouth.

> ### CAUTIONS FOR TOPICAL ORAL PROTECTANTS
> - Products containing glycyrrhiza (licorice) extract may affect blood pressure. Avoid concurrent use in patients with hypertension and those taking antihypertensive medications.
> - Products containing glycyrrhiza (licorice) extract cause induction of cytochrome P450 2C9 and 3A4. This may decrease levels of warfarin. Avoid concurrent use of warfarin and any drug that is a substrate of either 2C9 or 3A4.

- Oral Rinses
  - Active ingredients include eucalyptol, menthol, methyl salicylate, thymol, or bee propolis.
  - Adverse effects include soft tissue irritation and a bad taste in the mouth.

> ### CAUTIONS FOR ORAL RINSES
> - Eucalyptol may be associated with hypoglycemia. Avoid in patients with diabetes taking hypoglycemic agents.
> - Bee propolis can inhibit platelet aggregation. Although systemic absorption is limited or negligible, patients taking anticoagulant or antiplatelet medications should avoid this product.

Other Treatment Considerations

- *Pain, discomfort, and irritation* associated with RAS may also be treated with systemic analgesics (e.g., acetaminophen, ibuprofen, or naproxen).
  - Aspirin should never be retained in the mouth before swallowing nor placed in the area of an oral lesion, as it can cause a chemical burn with associated tissue damage.

Special Populations

- Pregnancy
  - No adequate and well-controlled studies have been conducted in pregnant women.
  - Pregnant patients should consult a dentist along with their OB/GYN before considering use of any oral debriding and wound-cleansing agents, topical oral anesthetics, topical oral protectants, or oral rinses.

- Breastfeeding
    - It is unknown how these products affect breastfeeding women.

- Pediatric Patients
    - These products are not FDA approved for use in pediatric populations and should not be used.

- Geriatric Patients
    - There are no special considerations for use of these products in older adult patients.

■ ● QuES❶: Talk with the patient

● *Patient Education/Counseling*

- Nonpharmacologic Talking Points
    - Avoid spicy or acidic foods until the lesions heal.
    - Avoid sharp-textured foods that may cause increased trauma to the lesion.
    - If desired, apply ice directly to the lesions in 10-minute increments but for no longer than 20 minutes in a given hour.
    - Do not use heat. If an infection is present, heat may spread the infection.
    - Because stress may play a role in the development of RAS, relaxation and stress removal may be useful and have shown reduction in ulcer frequency.
    - Patients with nutritional deficiencies that may serve as a contributing factor for the development of RAS should increase consumption of foods high in the deficient nutrients or take appropriate nutritional supplements.

- Pharmacologic Talking Points
    - Nonprescription medications provide symptomatic relief of RAS, but they do not prevent its recurrence.
    - Gels are the preferred drug delivery mode because they are easy to apply and less likely to be washed away by saliva.
    - Do not swallow these products.
    - Oral Debriding and Wound-Cleansing Agents
        - Apply after meals up to 4 times daily.
        - Do not use longer than 7 days.

- Topical Oral Anesthetics
  - These products may numb the mouth and tongue. If these effects occur, do not eat or drink until they go away.
- Topical Oral Protectants
  - Apply these products as needed, often 3–4 times daily.
  - Products available as a patch or dissolving disc must be placed against the lesion for 10–20 seconds. Once the disc adheres to the lesion, the barrier is formed, and the disc will stay in place until dissolved.
- Oral Rinses
  - Rinse the mouth with a saline solution to soothe discomfort or to prepare the lesion for application of a topical medication. For saline solution, add 1–3 teaspoons of salt to 4–8 ounces of warm tap water.

- Suggest medical referral if any of the following occur:
  - Symptoms persist after 7 days of treatment with oral debriding or wound-cleansing agents.
  - Lesions do not heal within 14 days.
  - Symptoms worsen while nonprescription medications are being used.
  - Signs and symptoms of a bacterial infection develop (e.g., fever, rash, swelling).

Clinical Pearls

- Specific product selection may come down to patient preference.

- Patients with recurrent RAS should avoid using toothpaste that contains sodium lauryl sulfate, which may be irritating to the oral mucosa.

References

1. Albanese NP, Donaldson M. Orofacial Pain and Discomfort. In: Krinsky DL, Ferreri SP, Henstreet BA, Hume AL, Newton GD, Rollins CJ, Tietze KJ, eds. *Handbook of Nonprescription Drugs: An Interactive Approach to Self-Care*. Washington, DC: American Pharmacists Association; 2017:623–649.

COLDS

Miranda Wilhelm, PharmD
and Cortney M. Mospan, PharmD, BCACP, BCGP

For complete information about this topic, consult Chapter 11, "Colds and Allergy," written by Kelly L. Scolaro and published in the *Handbook of Nonprescription Drugs*, 19th Edition.[1]

Self-Care of Colds

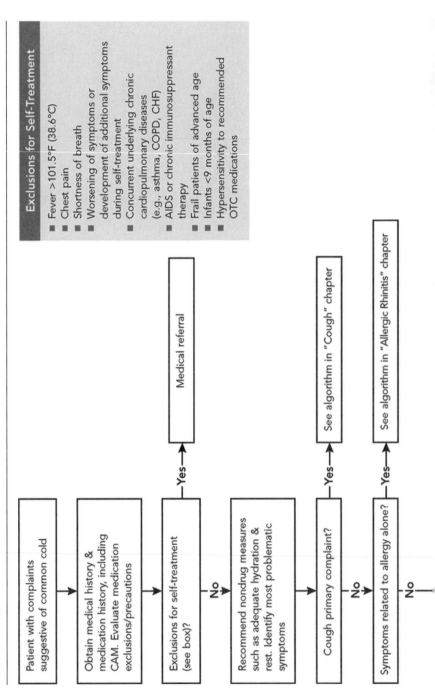

Exclusions for Self-Treatment

- Fever >101.5°F (38.6°C)
- Chest pain
- Shortness of breath
- Worsening of symptoms or development of additional symptoms during self-treatment
- Concurrent underlying chronic cardiopulmonary diseases (e.g., asthma, COPD, CHF)
- AIDS or chronic immunosuppressant therapy
- Frail patients of advanced age
- Infants <9 months of age
- Hypersensitivity to recommended OTC medications

Patient with complaints suggestive of common cold

↓

Obtain medical history & medication history, including CAM. Evaluate medication exclusions/precautions

↓

Exclusions for self-treatment (see box)? —Yes→ Medical referral

No ↓

Recommend nondrug measures such as adequate hydration & rest. Identify most problematic symptoms

↓

Cough primary complaint? —Yes→ See algorithm in "Cough" chapter

No ↓

Symptoms related to allergy alone? —Yes→ See algorithm in "Allergic Rhinitis" chapter

No ↓

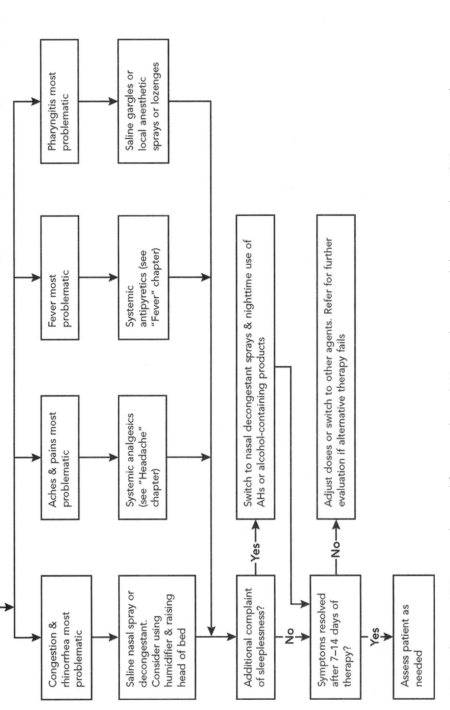

AH = antihistamine; AIDS = acquired immunodeficiency syndrome; CAM = complementary and alternative medicine; CHF = congestive heart failure; COPD = chronic obstructive pulmonary disorder; OTC = over-the-counter.

◨◨ Overview

- A cold, also known as the common cold, is a viral infection of the upper respiratory tract. More than 200 viruses cause colds, with the majority of colds in children and adults caused by rhinoviruses.

- Colds are usually self-limiting. There is no known cure.

- The goal of self-treatment is to reduce and manage bothersome symptoms.

◨◨ Pathophysiology

- Inside epithelial cells, the virus replicates and infection spreads to other cells. Peak viral concentrations occur 2–4 days after initial inoculation, and viruses are present in the nasopharynx for 16–18 days.

- Infected cells release distress signals that activate inflammatory mediators and neurogenic reflexes. These activation processes result in recruitment of additional inflammatory mediators, vasodilatation, transudation of plasma, and glandular secretion. This results in stimulation of pain nerve fibers and sneeze and cough reflexes.

- Inflammatory mediators and parasympathetic nervous system reflex mechanisms cause hypersecretion of watery nasal fluid. Cholinergic and sympathetic nerves are involved in congestion because they innervate glands and arteries that supply the glands. These will be targets for symptom management.

◨ Transmission

- The most efficient and common mode of viral transmission is self-inoculation of the nasal mucosa or conjunctiva after contact with viral-laden secretions on animate (e.g., hands) or inanimate (e.g., doorknobs and telephones) objects.

- Aerosol transmission is also common.

◨ Preventative Measures

- Proper hand hygiene reduces the transmission of cold viruses. Recommend the following strategies as accepted by and appropriate for the patient.
  - Frequent hand cleansing with soap and warm water for at least 20 seconds.
  - Alcohol-based hand sanitizers containing isopropanol or ethanol (60%-80% concentration).

- Chlorhexidine, povidone-iodine, and quaternary ammonium compounds are also effective alone or in combination with alcohol-based products.

■ Use of antiviral disinfectants such as Lysol (kills >99% of rhinoviruses after 1 minute) to clean inanimate objects and surfaces that may have been touched.

■ Antiviral tissues such as Kleenex Anti-Viral (tissue layer containing citric acid and sodium lauryl sulfate). Using plain facial tissues to cover mouth and nose when coughing or sneezing, and then promptly throwing them away.

■ ■ QuEST: Quickly and Accurate Assess the Patient Using SCHOLAR MAC

QuEST SCHOLAR is an acronym used to assess a patient to determine self-care candidate status and to identify which treatment would be most appropriate. See Chapter 1 for a description of the QuEST SCHOLAR process.

■ Does the Patient Have a Cold?

■ A predictable sequence of symptoms appears 1–3 days after infection.

■ Sore throat is the first symptom to appear.

■ Nasal symptoms dominate 2–3 days later. During the first 2 days of a cold, patients may report clear, thin, or watery nasal secretions, or combinations thereof. As the cold progresses, the secretions become thicker, and the color may change to yellow or green. When the cold begins to resolve, the secretions again become clear, thin, and/or watery.

■ Cough, although an infrequent symptom (<30%), appears by day 4 or 5.

■ Patients, especially children, may have low-grade fever, but colds are rarely associated with a fever above 100.4°F (38°C, oral).

■ Physical assessment of a patient with a cold may yield the following findings: slightly red pharynx with evidence of postnasal drainage, nasal obstruction, and mildly to moderately tender sinuses on palpation.

■ Rhinovirus cold symptoms persist for about 7–14 days.

■ See Table 1 for clinical presentation of other common respiratory disorders. These should be considered in the patient assessment.

TABLE 1. Differentiation of colds and other respiratory disorders

Illness	Signs and Symptoms
Allergic rhinitis	Watery eyes; itchy nose, eyes, or throat; repetitive sneezing; nasal congestion; watery rhinorrhea; red, irritated eyes with conjunctival injection
Asthma	Cough, dyspnea, wheezing
Bacterial throat infection	Sore throat (moderate-severe pain), fever, exudate, tender anterior cervical adenopathy
Colds	Sore throat (mild-moderate pain), nasal congestion, rhinorrhea, sneezing common, low-grade fever, chills, headache, malaise, myalgia, and cough possible
Croup	Fever, rhinitis, and pharyngitis initially, progressing to cough (may be "barking" cough), stridor, and dyspnea
Influenza	Myalgia, arthralgia, fever 100.4°F-102°F (38°C-38.9°C, oral), sore throat, nonproductive cough, moderate-severe fatigue
Otitis media	Ear popping, ear fullness, otalgia, otorrhea, hearing loss, dizziness
Pneumonia or bronchitis	Chest tightness, wheezing, dyspnea, productive cough, changes in sputum color, persistent fever
Sinusitis	Tenderness over the sinuses, facial pain aggravated by Valsalva maneuver or postural changes, fever above 101.5°F (38.6°C, oral), tooth pain, halitosis, upper respiratory tract symptoms for more than 7 days with poor response to decongestants
West Nile virus infection	Fever, headache, fatigue, rash, swollen lymph glands, and eye pain initially, possibly progressing to GI distress, CNS changes, seizures, or paralysis
Whooping cough	Initial catarrhal phase (rhinorrhea, mild cough, sneezing) of 1–2 weeks, followed by 1–6 weeks of paroxysmal coughing

▣ *Important SCHOLAR MAC Considerations*

■ Are symptoms more bothersome during a certain time of day? (e.g., trouble sleeping because of symptoms)

■ Is the patient experiencing nasal, sore throat, or cough symptoms, or all of these?
  ▪ Determine which symptom is the most bothersome to utilize single ingredient products as often as possible.
  ▪ Determine if sore throat is due to drainage (postnasal drip) running down the back of the throat to utilize first-generation antihistamines or pseudoephedrine.

▣ *Physical Assessment Techniques*

■ Observe the patient for signs of chronic medical conditions, such as red, watery eyes (allergic rhinitis); wheezing (asthma, chronic obstructive pulmonary disease [COPD]); productive cough (COPD); barrel chest (COPD); poorly perfused area (peripheral artery disease); enlarged lymph nodes (general infection); rash.

■ Obtain vital signs (e.g., temperature, respiratory rate, pulse, and blood pressure).

- Palpate sinuses and neck and observe any pain or tenderness.

- Visually examine throat for redness or exudates. If bacterial pharyngitis is suspected, run rapid strep test, if available.

- Auscultate chest to detect wheezing, crackles, and rapid or irregular heartbeat.

⬛ ⬛ QuⒺST: Establish that the patient is an appropriate self-care candidate

Utilize the information collected in the patient assessment with the treatment algorithm and exclusions for self-care to determine if self-care is appropriate.

⬛ Exclusions to Self-Care

Review the treatment algorithm and exclusions for self-care provided at the beginning of the chapter. This section highlights key exclusion criteria.

⬛ Medications

- Antihypertensives – potential treatment options can raise blood pressure, decreasing efficacy of blood pressure–lowering agents and increasing risk of adverse effects.

- Hypoglycemic agents – potential treatment options can affect insulin secretion, minimizing effects of hypoglygemic agents and elevating blood glucose.

- Selective Serotonin Reuptake Inhibitor (SSRI) and Selective Norepinephrine Reuptake Inhibitor (SNRI) – potential treatment options can have additive adrenergic stimulation, resulting in increased heart rate.

- Monoamine oxidase inhibitors (MAOI) – metabolism of potential treatment options can be decreased, leading to adverse effects. Concomitant use of decongestants and MAOIs should be avoided for 2 weeks after discontinuation.

- See Table 2 for a list of common drug interactions.

⬛ Conditions

- Hypertension, diabetes mellitus, hyperthyroidism, and benign prostatic hyperplasia could limit medication selection because of the drug-disease interactions and adverse effects.

TABLE 2. Clinically important drug-drug interactions with cold products

Drug/Drug Class	Potential Interaction (Drug-Specific Data)	Management/Prevention
Decongestants		
Ergot derivatives (e.g., dihydroergotamine and ergotamine)	Increased risk of hypertension and vasoconstriction	Avoid combination
Linezolid	Increased risk of hypertension	Reduce dose of decongestant and monitor closely. Consider therapy modification
MAOIs (e.g., phenelzine, selegiline)	Increased risk of hypertension	Avoid combination
Serotonin/norepinephrine reuptake inhibitors	Increased risk of tachycardia	Consider therapy modification
Antihistamines		
Anticholinergics (e.g., ipratropium, tiotropium, umeclidinium)	Enhanced anticholinergic effects (dry mouth, eyes, urinary retention, sedation)	Avoid combination
Brexpiprazole	Increased risk of brexpiprazole toxicity (diphenhydramine)	Reduce brexpiprazole by 25% or avoid combination
CNS depressants (alcohol, opiates, sedatives)	Increased sedation (sedating antihistamines, cetirizine)	Avoid combination
Metoprolol	Increased metoprolol serum concentrations and risk of hypotension (diphenhydramine)	Reduce metoprolol dose or avoid combination
Phenytoin	Decreased phenytoin elimination (chlorpheniramine)	Monitor therapy or avoid combination
Potassium chloride (oral)	Increased risk of ulcers	Avoid combination

- Other conditions associated with adrenergic stimulation may be worsened (e.g., heart disease, elevated intraocular pressure, ischemic heart disease).

- Nicotine users may also experience adverse effects because of the additive vasoconstriction with potential treatment options.

Special Populations

- Infants 3 months of age or younger should be referred because they cannot sufficiently clear mucus secretions.

- Frail older adults may not be appropriate candidates for self-care; all non-prescription medications should be considered for appropriateness and dose adjustments made as needed.

- Aspirin-containing products should not be used in children less than 16 years of age with viral illnesses because of the risk of Reye's syndrome.

■ ■ QuE⑤T: Suggest appropriate self-care strategies

Select the appropriate treatment option based on the previously collected patient data. Various treatment options are discussed along with clinical pearls and pertinent patient considerations for optimal management.

● Treatment Options

Nasal congestion treatment of choice is systemic or topical adrenergic agonist decongestants.

- Oral Decongestants
  - Pseudoephedrine is the oral decongestant of choice.
  - The efficacy of the current FDA-approved dose of phenylephrine has been highly debated. A study published in 2015 by Meltzer et al. showed phenylephrine was not more effective than a placebo in treating nasal congestion related to allergic rhinitis.[2]
  - Adverse effects associated with decongestants include cardiovascular stimulation (e.g., elevated blood pressure, tachycardia, palpitation, or arrhythmias) and central nervous system (CNS) stimulation (e.g., restlessness, insomnia, anxiety, tremors, fear, or hallucinations).

> **CAUTIONS FOR ORAL DECONGESTANTS**
> - Patients with hypertension should use systemic decongestants only with medical advice.
> - Decongestants are contraindicated in patients receiving concomitant MAOIs for 2 weeks after discontinuation.
> - Persons taking SSRI or SNRI antidepressants should use decongestants with caution, as these medications may increase heart rate.

- Topical Decongestants
  - Because of the limited systemic absorption, topical decongestants may be the preferred treatment option for special populations and patients with comorbidities.
  - Therapy should be limited to 3–5 days in duration to avoid rhinitis medicamentosa (rebound congestion). However, some studies show that durations of 10 days to 8 weeks appear to be safe.
  - Aromatic oil (camphor, menthol, and eucalyptus) products such as Vicks VapoRub (ages ≥ 2 years) ease nasal congestion and improve sleep by producing a soothing sensation.

> **CAUTIONS FOR TOPICAL DECONGESTANTS**
> - Patients with hypertension should use topical decongestants cautiously.

- Nonpharmacologic Options
  - Medical devices such as Breathe Right nasal strips lift the nares open, thus enlarging the anterior nasal passages.

Rhinorrhea treatment of choice is a first-generation ("sedating") antihistamine. Second-generation antihistamines are not effective for the treatment of colds.

- Benefit may be seen in adults if used early in the course of a cold (e.g., day 1 or 2 of symptom onset).

- Combination therapy with first-generation antihistamines and decongestants showed some benefit in adults, but the significance of the data is questionable.

- Adverse effects associated with first-generation antihistamines may include dry mouth and throat, constipation, blurred vision, urinary retention, and tinnitus.

> **CAUTIONS FOR FIRST-GENERATION ("SEDATING") ANTIHISTAMINES**
> - Before used in the management of the cold, should determine if potential benefits outweigh known risks associated with these drugs.
> - First-generation antihistamines are contraindicated in prostatic hyperplasia and angle-closure glaucoma.
> - Children tend to be more sensitive to CNS excitatory effects, while adults are more likely to experience CNS depression.
> - First-generation antihistamines are listed as Potentially Inappropriate Medications for Older Adults in the 2015 American Geriatrics Society (AGS) Beers Criteria. The AGS recommends avoiding use in older adults. Use in patients with dementia may worsen cognitive decline.

Pharyngitis can be treated with local anesthetics and systemic analgesics.

- Lozenges or sprays containing benzocaine or dyclonine hydrochloride may be used every 2–4 hours.

- Emerging evidence suggests that menthol and camphor may be effective.

- Local antiseptics (e.g., cetylpyridinium chloride or hexylresorcinol) are **not** effective for viral infections.

- Sucking on hard candy, gargling with salt water (1/2 to 1 teaspoon of salt per 8 ounces of warm water), or drinking fruit juices or hot tea with lemon may ease sore throats.

CAUTIONS FOR LOCAL ANESTHETICS

- Patients with a history of allergic reactions to anesthetics should avoid products with benzocaine.
- Benzocaine has been associated with methemoglobinemia and should be avoided in children less than 2 years of age. Seek medical attention if any of the following occur after using benzocaine products: pale, gray- or blue-colored skin, lips, and nail beds; headache; light-headedness; shortness of breath; fatigue; and rapid heart rate.

◼ Other Treatment Considerations

- *Pain and fever* sometimes associated with colds can be effectively treated with systemic analgesics (e.g., acetaminophen, ibuprofen, or naproxen).

- *Cough* associated with colds is usually nonproductive.
    - The use of antitussives (codeine or dextromethorphan) has questionable efficacy in colds and is not recommended.
    - Guaifenesin, an expectorant, has not been proven effective in natural colds.

- Although evidence of efficacy is lacking, popular general treatment measures include increased fluid intake, adequate rest, nutritious diet as tolerated, and increased humidification with steamy showers, vaporizers, or humidifiers.

- Saline nasal sprays or drops moisten irritated mucosal membranes and loosen encrusted mucus. (See Appendix 1 for administration guidelines.)

◼ Complementary Therapy

T3 See Table 3 for selected botanical natural products marketed for the treatment of colds.

- Oral zinc (lozenges or syrup) was effective in reducing cold symptoms and duration if started within 24 hours of symptom onset and administered

TABLE 3. Selected complementary therapies for colds

Agent	Risks	Effectiveness
Botanical Natural Products (Scientific Name)		
African geranium (umckaloabo, active ingredient in Umcka ColdCare products [*Pelargonium sidoides*])	Allergic reactions or GI disturbances	Some evidence for alleviating symptoms of acute rhinosinusitis associated with colds in adults
Ephedra (ma huang [*Ephedra sinica*])	Tachycardia, hypertension, heart attack, stroke, seizure	Effective decongestant
Goldenseal (*Hydrastis canadensis*)	Potentially toxic, especially in patients with glucose-6-dehydrogenase deficiency	Some evidence of anti-inflammatory effects of active ingredient berberine for treatment of pulmonary inflammation

every 2 hours while awake. The study also reported prophylaxis with zinc for at least 5 months reduced the incidence of colds in healthy patients. Nasal formulations have been removed from the market because of anosmia (loss of smell) associated with their use.

■ Routine use of high-dose vitamin C (≥2 g/day) does not appear to prevent colds in the general population but does reduce the duration mildly. Vitamin C taken after the onset of a cold is not effective in reducing symptom duration or severity. High-dose vitamin C prophylaxis is effective in preventing colds in patients subjected to severe physical stress (e.g., marathon runners). Doses of 4 g/day or more are associated with gastrointestinal (GI) symptoms and should not be recommended.

■ Products that claim to strengthen the immune system such as Airborne, Emergen-C Immune+, etc. are available but have not been proven to be effective in preventing or treating colds.

■ Special Populations

■ Pregnancy
- ■ Because most colds are self-limiting with bothersome rather than life-threatening symptoms, nonpharmacologic therapy is preferred. Saline nasal spray is a safe option to provide congestion relief.
- ■ Most of the active ingredients in FDA-approved cold medications are Pregnancy Risk Category B or C. Systemic decongestants theoretically decrease fetal blood flow and should be avoided. Oral phenylephrine during the first trimester has been associated with minor malformations (e.g., inguinal hernia, hip dislocation). Pseudoephedrine has been linked to abdominal wall defects (gastroschisis) in newborns.

Oxymetazoline is poorly absorbed after intranasal administration and is the preferred topical decongestant during pregnancy.

■ Breastfeeding

- The American Academy of Pediatrics has found pseudoephedrine to be compatible with breastfeeding. Because decongestants may decrease milk production, lactating mothers should monitor their milk production and drink extra fluids as needed.
- No human data are available for intranasal phenylephrine and oxymetazoline, so they are considered "probably compatible" in lactating mothers. Therefore, pseudoephedrine is the preferred decongestant in breastfeeding mothers.
- Dextromethorphan, guaifenesin, benzocaine, camphor (topical), and menthol (topical) have low risks of birth defects and have been found to be compatible with breastfeeding.

■ Pediatric Patients

- Using nonprescription cold products in children is controversial owing to the lack of clinical evidence of safety and efficacy in this age group.
- FDA does not recommend nonprescription cold medications for children younger than 2 years because of the lack of efficacy and risk of misuse or overuse, leading to adverse events and death. Manufacturers have voluntarily updated product labeling to include the statement, "Do not use in children under four years of age," and added warnings to antihistamine-containing products against their use for sedation purposes.
- Nondrug measures for infants and children include upright positioning to enhance nasal drainage, maintaining fluid intake, increasing the humidity of inspired air, and irrigating the nose with saline drops.
- Children typically cannot blow their own noses until about 4 years of age; carefully clearing the nasal passageways with a bulb syringe may be necessary if accumulation of mucus interferes with sleeping or eating.

■ Geriatric Patients

- Older adults are more likely than other age groups to experience adverse effects with systemic decongestant use.
- Decongestants interact with numerous drugs, so older adults taking multiple medications should be encouraged to ask their pharmacist before taking nonprescription medications.

■ ■ QuES❶: Talk with the patient

■ *Patient Education/Counseling*

- Nonpharmacologic Talking Points
    - Upright positioning and use of nasal bulb syringe are first-line strategies in infants and children who are not eligible for pharmacologic therapy.

- Pharmacologic Talking Points
    - Systemic Decongestants
        - Avoid taking dose at bedtime because of the adverse effects of insomnia and restlessness.
        - Patients who use systemic decongestants with comorbidities should be instructed to closely monitor for adverse effects (e.g., palpitations, elevated blood pressure, and elevated blood glucose).
        - The maximum dose of pseudoephedrine is 240 mg daily.
    - Topical Decongestants
        - The patient should not use topical decongestants longer than 3–5 days because of the risk for rebound congestion.
    - Local Anesthetics
        - Benzocaine and dyclonine may numb the mouth and tongue. If these effects occur, do not eat or drink until they go away.
    - First-Generation ("Sedating") Antihistamines
        - The patient should be counseled to limit daytime use of antihistamines because of the questionable benefit and risk of sedation.

- Suggest medical referral if any of the following occur:
    - Symptoms last longer than 7 to 14 days.
    - Sore throat persists more than several days, is severe, or is associated with persistent fever, headache, or nausea or vomiting.
    - Symptoms worsen while nonprescription medications are being taken.
    - Signs and symptoms of a bacterial infection develop (e.g., thick nasal or respiratory secretions that are not clear, temperature higher than 101.5°F [38.6°C, oral], shortness of breath, chest congestion, wheezing, rash, or significant ear pain).

■ *Clinical Pearls*

- In managing cold symptoms, always look at the patient in front of you. If the patient has comorbidities (e.g., diabetes or hypertension) but is well-controlled, the risk of a short course of decongestant use is likely not significant. Greater concern exists in patients with unmanaged or undiagnosed conditions.

■ Select single-entity products as much as possible, even if this requires the use of two or three products. Treatment should be directed at the most bothersome symptom(s). Only recommend combination products to the patient when all ingredients are indicated for symptom management.

⬛⬤ References

1. Scolaro K. Colds and allergy. In: Krinsky DL, Ferreri SP, Henstreet BA, Hume AL, Newton GD, Rollins CJ, Tietze KJ, eds. *Handbook of Nonprescription Drugs: An Interactive Approach to Self-Care*. Washington, DC: American Pharmacists Association; 2017:189–216.

2. Meltzer EO, Ratner PH, McGraw T. Oral phenylephrine HCL for nasal congestion in seasonal allergic rhinitis: A randomized, open-label, placebo-controlled study. *J Allergy Clin Immunol Pract*. 2015 Sep-Oct;3(5):702–708.

3. American Geriatrics Society 2015 Beers Criteria Update Expert Panel. American Geriatrics Society 2015 updated beers criteria for potentially inappropriate medication use in older adults. *J Am Geriatr Soc*. 2015;63(11):2227–2246.

CONSTIPATION

Cortney M. Mospan, PharmD, BCACP, BCGP

For complete information about this topic, consult Chapter 15, "Constipation," written by Kristin W. Weitzel and Jean-Venable "Kelly" R. Goode and published in the *Handbook of Nonprescription Drugs*, 19th Edition.[1]

Self-Care of Constipation

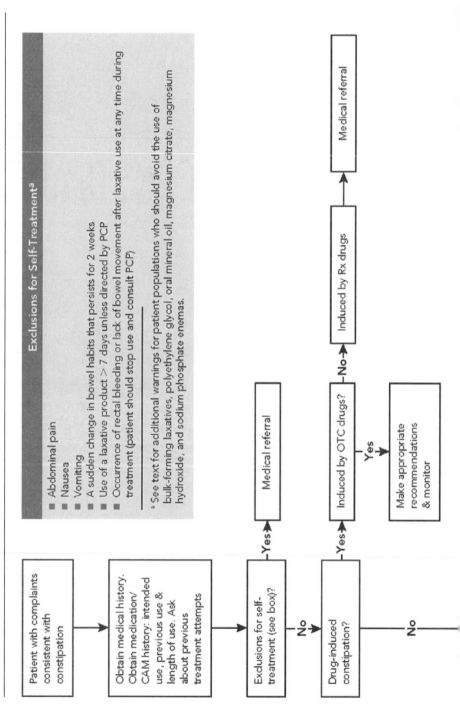

Patient with complaints consistent with constipation

↓

Obtain medical history. Obtain medication/ CAM history: intended use, previous use & length of use. Ask about previous treatment attempts

↓

Exclusions for self-treatment (see box)? —Yes→ Medical referral

↓ No

Drug-induced constipation? —Yes→ Induced by OTC drugs? —Yes→ Make appropriate recommendations & monitor

↓ No

—No→ Induced by Rx drugs → Medical referral

Exclusions for Self-Treatment[a]

- Abdominal pain
- Nausea
- Vomiting
- A sudden change in bowel habits that persists for 2 weeks
- Use of a laxative product > 7 days unless directed by PCP
- Occurrence of rectal bleeding or lack of bowel movement after laxative use at any time during treatment (patient should stop use and consult PCP)

[a] See text for additional warnings for patient populations who should avoid the use of bulk-forming laxatives, polyethylene glycol, oral mineral oil, magnesium citrate, magnesium hydroxide, and sodium phosphate enemas.

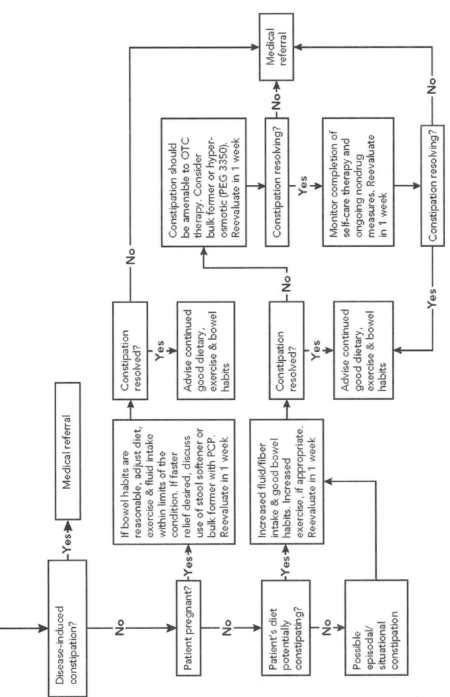

CAM = complementary and alternative medicine; OTC = over-the-counter; PCP = primary care provider; PEG = polyethylene glycol; Rx = prescription.

■ ■ Overview

- Bowel habits and frequency vary, but constipation is generally defined as fewer than 3 bowel movements per week with straining or difficult passage of hard, dry stools, or both.

- Older adult patients, women, late-term pregnancy, and post-childbirth are populations most likely to experience constipation.

- If left untreated, constipation can lead to development of anal fissures, hemorrhoids, rectal prolapse, fecal impaction, and other complications.

- The goal of self-treatment is to relieve constipation while reestablishing normal bowel habits and preventing future episodes.

■ ■ Pathophysiology

- Following ingestion, food is partially digested in the stomach and then moved to the duodenum via peristaltic waves. Contractions continue to move food through the intestines; the defecation process involves both voluntary and involuntary reflexes.

- Constipation causes include medical problems, medications, physiologic and psychological disturbances (e.g., menopause, dehydration, stress), and lifestyle characteristics (e.g., low fiber diet, lack of exercise).

- Failing to heed the urge to empty the bowels can lead to constipation.

■ ■ QuEST: Quickly and Accurate Assess the Patient Using SCHOLAR MAC

QuEST SCHOLAR is an acronym used to assess a patient to determine self-care candidate status and to identify which treatment would be most appropriate. See Chapter 1 for a description of the QuEST SCHOLAR process.

■ Is the Patient Experiencing Constipation?

- Patients should report a decreased frequency or difficulty passing stools compared to what is normal for them.

■ Additional symptoms can include dull headache, abdominal discomfort, bloating, flatulence, lower back pain, anorexia, lassitude, and psychosocial distress.

● Important SCHOLAR MAC Considerations

■ What frequency and consistency of bowel movements is "normal" for the patient?

■ What are the characteristics of the patient's bowel movements (caliber, color, texture)?

■ How long has the patient been experiencing constipation?
  ▪ Occasional bouts lasting less than 7 days are treatable with self-care measures.
  ▪ Constipation that lasts several weeks or months or that is associated with concomitant conditions requires therapy beyond the self-care approach.

■ How soon does the patient need or want relief?
  ▪ Determine if the patient needs immediate relief because of discomfort (<12 hours) or if they are seeking treatment for prevention of constipation or regulation of their bowel habits.

■ What is the underlying cause of constipation?
  ▪ Does the patient have a diet that may be contributing to constipation?
  ▪ Does the patient have a disease state that may be contributing to constipation?

■ Has the patient been passing gas?
  ▪ **Lack of gas may signal an obstruction.**

■ ■ QuEST: Establish that the patient is an appropriate self-care candidate

Utilize the information collected in the patient assessment with the treatment algorithm and exclusions for self-care to determine if self-care is appropriate.

● Exclusions to Self-Care

Review the treatment algorithm and exclusions for self-care provided at the beginning of the chapter. This section highlights key exclusion criteria.

◉ Medications

- Patients using laxatives daily, excluding fiber-based therapies, should see a primary care provider.

- The patient's prescription medications, nonprescription medications, and dietary supplements should be reviewed for potential association, and therapies should be adjusted if possible.

- See Table 1 for a list of medications that may cause constipation.

- See Table 2 for a list of common drug interactions.

◉ Conditions

- Patients with paraplegia, quadriplegia, irritable bowel syndrome, inflammatory bowel disease, and colostomy should be referred to their primary care provider, as underlying disease factors may need to be addressed.

- Patients experiencing blood in their stools or black, tarry stools should be referred.

- Patients with significant changes in bowel habits and accompanying weight loss should not be treated with self-care measures.

◉ Special Populations

- Children less than two years of age should be assessed by their pediatrician before utilizing nonprescription treatments.

TABLE 1. Selected drugs that may induce constipation

Analgesics (including nonsteroidal anti-inflammatory drugs)	Hematinics (especially iron)
Antacids (e.g., calcium and aluminum compounds, bismuth)	Hyperlipidemics (e.g., cholestyramine, pravastatin, simvastatin)
Anticholinergics (e.g., benztropine, glycopyrrolate)	Hypotensives (e.g., angiotensin-converting enzyme inhibitors, beta blockers)
Anticonvulsants (e.g., carbamazepine, divalproate)	Muscle relaxants (e.g., cyclobenzaprine, metaxalone)
Antidepressants (specifically, tricyclics such as amitriptyline)	Opiates (e.g., morphine, codeine)
Antihistamines (e.g., diphenhydramine, loratadine)	Parkinsonism agents (e.g., bromocriptine)
Antimuscarinics (e.g., oxybutynin, tolterodine)	Polystyrene sodium sulfonate
Benzodiazepines (especially alprazolam and estazolam)	Psychotherapeutic drugs (e.g., phenothiazines, butyrophenones)
Calcium channel blockers (e.g., verapamil, diltiazem)	Sedative hypnotics (e.g., zolpidem, benzodiazepines, phenobarbital)
Calcium supplements (e.g., calcium carbonate)	Serotonin agonists (e.g., ondansetron)
Diuretics (e.g., hydrochlorothiazide, furosemide)	Sucralfate

TABLE 2. Clinically important drug-drug interactions with nonprescription laxative agents

Laxative Agent	Drug	Potential Interaction	Management/ Preventive Measures
Bulk-forming laxatives (e.g., psyllium)	Digoxin, anticoagulants, salicylates, and potentially other oral drugs	Interference with drug absorption	Separate dosing of prescription oral medications by at least 2 hours
Docusate salts	Mineral oil	Increased absorption of mineral oil	Avoid concurrent use
Magnesium citrate	Fluoroquinolone and tetracycline antibiotics	Decreased drug absorption	Avoid oral magnesium citrate within 1 to 3 hours of oral tetracyclines or fluoroquinolones
Magnesium hydroxide	Captopril, cefdinir, some oral bisphosphonates, gabapentin, iron salts, nitrofurantoin, phenothiazines, phenytoin, rosuvastatin	Decreased oral bioavailability, rate or extent of drug absorption, or combinations thereof	Separate dosing by at least 2 hours for most agents
Magnesium hydroxide	Ketoconazole, itraconazole, fluoroquinolone and tetracycline antibiotics, levothyroxine	Decreased drug absorption	Avoid magnesium hydroxide for at least 4 hours before or up to 3 hours after interacting agent
Bisacodyl	Milk products or drugs that raise gastric pH (e.g., proton pump inhibitors)	Premature dissolution of the bisacodyl enteric coating, leading to gastric irritation or dyspepsia	Avoid milk products or interacting drugs within 1 hour before or after bisacodyl

■ ■ QuEST: Suggest appropriate self-care strategies

Select the appropriate treatment option based on the previously collected patient data. Various treatment options are discussed along with clinical pearls and pertinent patient considerations for optimal management.

■ Treatment Options

Prevention of constipation treatment of choice is bulk-forming laxatives. Hyperosmotic agents and emollients may also be used.

- Bulk-Forming Laxatives
    - This class includes methylcellulose, psyllium, and polycarbophil.
    - These are recommended in most cases of constipation because their mechanism of action most closely approximates the natural physiologic process to produce a bowel movement.
    - These agents are useful in patients who should avoid straining (e.g., following heart attack, childbirth) and in patients with low-fiber diets.

TABLE 3. Classification of laxatives

Bulk-Forming Laxatives	Stimulant Laxatives	Saline Laxatives
Calcium polycarbophil, methylcellulose, psyllium	Sennosides, bisacodyl	Magnesium citrate, magnesium hydroxide, dibasic sodium phosphate, monobasic sodium phosphate, magnesium sulfate
Hyperosmotic Laxatives	**Emollient Laxatives**	**Lubricant Laxatives**
PEG 3350, glycerin	Docusate sodium, docusate calcium	Mineral oil

- Onset of action is 12–24 hours but can take up to 72 hours.
- Bulk-forming laxatives can interfere with drug absorption and should be separated by 2 hours from other medications.
- Adverse effects are minimal when used as directed, but abdominal cramping and flatulence are most common.

CAUTIONS FOR BULK-FORMING LAXATIVES

- If not taken with at least 8 oz. of fluid, these can swell in the throat, causing choking.
- These should be avoided in patients with swallowing difficulties or esophageal strictures, intestinal ulcerations, stenosis, or disabling adhesions.
- Patients with fluid restrictions (e.g., heart failure) may need to avoid.

- Hyperosmotic Agents
  - This class includes polyethylene glycol 3350 (PEG 3350).
  - Onset of action is 12–72 hours but may take as long as 96 hours.
  - No clinically significant drug interactions have been reported.
  - Adverse effects are limited but can include abdominal discomfort, cramping, bloating, and flatulence.

CAUTIONS FOR HYPEROSMOTIC LAXATIVES

- Patients with renal disease or irritable bowel syndrome should seek primary care provider approval before use.

- Emollients (Stool Softeners)
  - This class includes docusate sodium and docusate calcium. There is no clinical difference between the sodium and calcium salts.

- These are best used to in patients who should avoid straining (e.g., recent abdominal surgery, hemorrhoids, recent myocardial infarction, postpartum) or in patients with painful defecation.
- Onset of action is 12–72 hours but can take 3–5 days to see effect.
- Docusate is not appreciably absorbed from the gastrointestinal (GI) tract and does not hamper absorption of other medications.
- Adverse effects are rare unless larger-than-recommended doses are taken; weakness, sweating, muscle cramps, and irregular heartbeat can occur.

CAUTIONS FOR EMOLLIENTS

- Do not take with mineral oil.

Acute relief of constipation treatment of choice is saline laxatives, or hyperosmotic laxatives.

- Saline Laxatives
    - This class includes magnesium citrate, magnesium hydroxide, dibasic sodium phosphate, monobasic sodium phosphate, and magnesium sulfate.
    - Oral magnesium hydroxide is the treatment of choice for occasional acute relief of constipation in otherwise healthy patients. A bowel movement will occur within 30 minutes-6 hours.
    - Other products (e.g., magnesium citrate) can be used for colonoscopy prep. A bowel movement will occur within 30 minutes-3 hours for oral doses and 2–15 minutes for rectal doses.
    - No more than one nonprescription sodium phosphate product should be used in a 24-hour period. Appendix 1 provides administration techniques for rectal enemas.
    - Adverse effects include abdominal cramping, nausea, vomiting, and dehydration. If used long-term or at doses higher than recommended, electrolyte imbalances can occur.

CAUTIONS FOR SALINE LAXATIVES

- Magnesium-containing laxatives should be avoided in patients on sodium-, phosphate-, or magnesium-restricted diets.
- Magnesium-containing laxatives should be avoided in individuals at high risk for magnesium toxicity (newborns, older adults, renal impairment).

- Sodium phosphate–containing products should be used cautiously in patients with renal impairment, on sodium-restricted diets, and taking medications that can affect electrolyte levels (e.g., diuretics).
- Sodium phosphate products are contraindicated in patients with heart failure.
- Rectally administered sodium phosphate products should be avoided in patients with megacolon, GI obstruction, imperforate anus, or colostomy.

- Hyperosmotic Laxatives
  - This class includes glycerin suppositories for acute relief of constipation.
  - Onset of action is 15–30 minutes to stimulate a bowel movement.
  - Glycerin suppositories are safe for use in patients 2 years of age and older, but with different adult and pediatric doses.
  - Adverse effects are limited but can include rectal irritation.

CAUTIONS FOR EMOLLIENT LAXATIVES

- Rectal irritation is possible with overdosage and should be avoided in patients with pre-existing rectal irritation.

- Lubricant Laxatives
  - Mineral oil is the only nonprescription lubricant, but the risks generally outweigh benefits of use.
  - Onset of action is 6–8 hours after oral administration and 5–15 minutes after rectal administration.
  - Adverse effects include impaired absorption of fat-soluble vitamins (ADEK), oil leakage, pruritus, crypititis, or other perianal conditions.

CAUTIONS FOR LUBRICANT LAXATIVES

- After an oral dose, patients should not lay down because of the risk of lipid pneumonia from aspiration. There is a warning for use in patients less than 6 years old, pregnant women, bedridden patients, older adults, and individuals with swallowing difficulties.

Opioid-induced constipation treatment of choice is stimulant laxatives.

■ Stimulant Laxatives
  ▪ This class includes sennosides, bisacodyl, and castor oil.
  ▪ Combination products, including docusate (stool softener), are often used for synergistic benefits.
  ▪ Onset of action for oral products is generally 6–10 hours but may take up to 24 hours. Bisacodyl suppositories usually produce a bowel movement within 15–60 minutes.
  ▪ Adverse effects include electrolyte and fluid deficiencies, enteric loss of protein, malabsorption, severe cramping, and hypokalemia. Sennosides can also cause urine discoloration.

> **CAUTIONS FOR STIMULANT LAXATIVES**
>
> ▪ Overdoses require prompt medical attention; symptoms include nausea, diarrhea, sudden vomiting, and severe abdominal cramping.
> ▪ High dosages can cause cramping, increased mucus secretion, and excessive evacuation of fluid.

■ Complementary Therapy
  ▪ Wheat dextrin, powdered cellulose, inulin, and partially hydrolyzed guar gum are dietary supplement products that can be used as fiber supplements.
  ▪ Aloe vera stimulant laxative and cascara products remain available, despite being banned for use by the FDA, since they are not considered GRAS (generally recognized as safe). Patients interested should be informed of the lack of proven safety, and the products should not be recommended.
  ▪ Flaxseed can also be recommended for constipation management. A double-blind trial found flaxseed superior to psyllium in decreasing constipation, bloating, and abdominal pain over 3 months in patients with irritable bowel syndrome. Overall, there is a large body of evidence to support psyllium's effectiveness; health care providers should carefully consider flaxseed's utility compared to other standards of care in nonprescription constipation treatment.
  ▪ Probiotics are an emerging area of interest for constipation treatment. They are thought to treat constipation by altering GI flora, stimulating motility and peristalsis, accelerating gut transit, or combinations

thereof. A systematic review of 5 randomized controlled trials has suggested potential benefit, but overall efficacy and clinical relevance of study outcomes were questioned. Information on Common Probiotics is available in Appendix 6.

Special Populations

Pregnancy

- Constipation is common in pregnancy, and dietary measures (e.g., increasing fluids and fiber intake) are first-line.
- Laxatives should be added only after nondrug approaches are determined insufficient. Bulk-forming laxatives are recommended initially with additional fluid intake. Alternatively, some health care providers recommend PEG 3350 first-line because of the low systemic absorption.
- Docusate can be used for patients with primarily dry, hard stools.
- Short-term bisacodyl or sennosides use is considered low-risk. Some health care providers prefer these agents because of greater availability of data for use in pregnancy.
- Castor oil, mineral oil, and saline laxatives should be avoided because they have greater risks than other therapies. Castor oil has been associated with uterine contraction and rupture. Saline laxatives can cause electrolyte imbalances.

Breastfeeding

- Laxatives can be used postpartum to reestablish normal bowel function; docusate is frequently used immediately following delivery to minimize straining.
- Sennosides, bisacodyl, PEG 3350, and docusate are considered compatible with breastfeeding, as they are minimally absorbed or do not accumulate in significant concentration in breast milk.
- Castor oil and mineral oil should be avoided.

Pediatric Patients

- Before recommending a laxative product, possible causes should be identified and addressed if possible. Common causes in children include unavailability of toilet facilities, chronic medical conditions, emotional distress, febrile illness, fear of defecation, pain from straining or stool passage, family conflict, and change in daily routine or environment.
- Mild constipation can often be relieved with dietary or behavioral

modifications (e.g., increased intake of sorbitol-containing fruit juices).

- Nonprescription products approved in children ages 2–6 include docusate sodium, magnesium hydroxide, and sennosides. Rectal use of glycerin, mineral oil, and sodium phosphate products are also approved.
- If occasional relief is needed, oral docusate or magnesium hydroxide are first-line. If faster relief is needed, pediatric glycerin suppositories can be recommended in children ages 2–6.
- Nonprescription products approved for children ages 6–12 include methylcellulose, calcium polycarbophil, psyllium powder, docusate sodium, mineral oil, magnesium citrate, magnesium hydroxide, magnesium sulfate, sennosides, bisacodyl, and castor oil. PEG 3350 is not approved for use in children younger than 17 years of age, but pediatricians frequently will recommend use. Rectal use of glycerin suppositories, mineral oil, sodium phosphate, and bisacodyl are also approved.
- In children ages 6–12, bulk-forming agents, docusate sodium, or magnesium hydroxide should be recommended first-line; oral stimulants are reserved for when these fail.
- Magnesium sulfate and castor oil are not recommended despite approval in some ages, as safer agents are available.

- **Geriatric Patients**
    - Older adult patients are at a greater risk of constipation because of dietary changes, decreased physical activity, comorbid conditions, use of medications that cause constipation, and physiologic changes.
    - A comprehensive medication review should be conducted when assessing constipation symptoms.
    - Lifestyle modifications are first-line therapy, but these must be considered in the context of comorbid conditions (e.g., increasing water intake in patients with congestive heart failure).
    - If lifestyle interventions are ineffective, bulk-forming laxatives are appropriate as a first-line laxative. If these cannot be used, do not provide sufficient relief, or a faster onset of action is desired, PEG 3350 is also acceptable to use.
    - Mineral oil should be avoided because of aspiration pneumonia risk, and saline laxatives should be avoided because of risk of electrolyte imbalances.
    - Rectal enemas may be appropriate if fecal impaction is suspected, but sodium phosphate products need to be used with caution.

◼ ◼ QuES❶: Talk with the patient

◼ Patient Education/Counseling

- ◼ Nonpharmacologic Talking Points
    - ▪ A balanced diet incorporating fruits, vegetables, and whole grains is key in preventing constipation. Added fiber normalizes frequency of bowel movements and GI transit, which decreases risk of excessive water reabsorption from stool, leading to dry, hard stools.
    - ▪ Patients with low fiber intake should gradually increase dietary intake of insoluble fiber (e.g., fruits, vegetables, wheat bran, whole grains) to minimize GI irritation. Goal is 25–35 grams of fiber a day.
    - ▪ When adding dietary fiber, patients should increase fluid intake by ~2 L/day.
    - ▪ Fiber dietary supplements can be used to increase fiber intake if dietary modifications are not sufficient.
    - ▪ Bowel training can promote bowel movements (reflexes are strongest first 30 minutes of day and after a meal).
    - ▪ Low physical activity levels have been associated with constipation.
    - ▪ Bowel habit frequency and patterns vary. Daily bowel movements are not a physical necessity, which can limit unnecessary laxative use.

- ◼ Pharmacologic Talking Points
    - ▪ Bulk-Forming Laxatives
        - ▫ Ensure these are mixed with at least 8 oz. of fluid for each dose to prevent intestinal blockage and that they are quickly consumed after mixing.
        - ▫ Patients with diabetes and other carbohydrate- or calorie-restricted diets should choose sugar-free formulations.
    - ▪ Hyperosmotic Laxatives
        - ▫ Ensure PEG 3350 is mixed in 4–8 oz. of a hot, cold, or room-temperature beverage (e.g., water, soda, juice, coffee, tea).
    - ▪ Saline Laxatives
        - ▫ Take each dose with 8 oz. of water to prevent dehydration, and do not exceed more than one dose in a 24-hour period.
    - ▪ Stimulant Laxatives
        - ▫ Enteric-coated bisacodyl can reduce gastric irritation, but these should not be broken, chewed, or given with anything that will increase gastric pH.
        - ▫ Enteric-coated or soft-gel formulations of bisacodyl should not be given within 1 hour of antacids, Histamine 2 Receptor

Antagonists (H2RAs), proton pump inhibitors (PPIs), or milk because of the rapid erosion of the enteric coating and potential for decreased effectiveness.[2]

- Suggest medical referral if any of the following occur:
  - Rectal bleeding occurs at any time.
  - Constipation persists despite therapy (>7 days).
  - Sudden change in bowel habits that persists for longer than 2 weeks.
  - Patients experience severe abdominal cramping, distention, fever, or other symptoms that may indicate a more serious condition (e.g., appendicitis).

Clinical Pearls

- Gritty, bulk-forming laxative powders can be mixed with orange juice or smoothies instead of water to improve texture and palatability.

- Generally, it is best to avoid taking laxatives within 2 hours of other medications to reduce the risk of decreased drug absorption because of the laxative effects.

- Patients should be assessed for medication history and medications with narrow therapeutic indices (e.g., digoxin, warfarin, sodium polystyrene sulfonate) to ensure there is a plan to monitor for serum drug level changes that may occur.

References

1. Weitzel KW, Goode JVR. In: Krinsky DL, Ferreri SP, Hemstreet, Hume AL, Newton GD, Rollins CJ, Tietze KJ, eds. *Handbook of Nonprescription Drugs: An Interactive Approach to Self-Care*. Washington, DC: American Pharmacists Association; 2017:265–285.

2. DailyMed. Womens gentle laxative- bisacodyl capsule, gelatin coated. https://dailymed.nlm.nih.gov/dailymed/drugInfo.cfm?setid=df96f688-e5d7-4a36-930b-e49ab1a8463f. Accessed June 12, 2018.

COUGH

Miranda Wilhelm, PharmD

For complete information about this topic, consult Chapter 12, "Cough," written by Karen Tietze and published in the *Handbook of Nonprescription Drugs, 19th Edition.*[1]

Self-Care of Cough

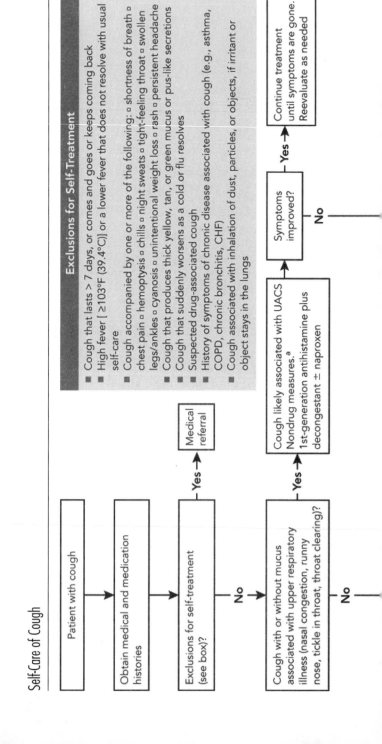

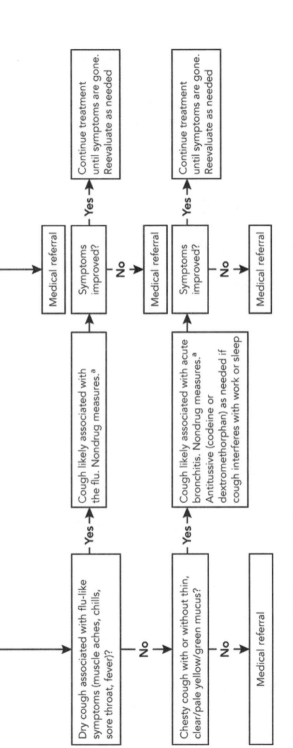

ª Nondrug measures: rest, fluids, vaporizer, and reassurance.

CHF = congestive heart failure; COPD = chronic obstructive pulmonary disease; UACS = upper airway cough syndrome.

⬛⬛ Overview

- Cough is the most common symptom for which patients seek medical care.

- The primary goal of self-treatment of cough is to reduce the number and severity of cough episodes. The second goal is to prevent complications. Cough treatment is symptomatic; the underlying disorder must be treated to stop the cough.

⬛⬛ Pathophysiology

- Cough is initiated by stimulation of chemically and mechanically sensitive, vagally mediated sensory pathways in the airway epithelium. A complex medullary brainstem network ("cough control center") processes the sensory input and stimulates the motor efferents. Viruses promote cough by a different, though not well understood, mechanism.

- Acute cough (≤3 weeks) is commonly caused by the common cold, acute bronchitis, pertussis, allergic rhinitis, aspiration syndromes, asthma and chronic obstructive pulmonary disease (COPD) exacerbations, pneumonia, pulmonary embolism, and acute left ventricular failure.

- Subacute cough (3–8 weeks) is commonly caused by infection.

- Chronic cough (≥8 weeks) is commonly caused by upper airway cough syndrome, asthma and COPD, gastroesophageal reflux disease (GERD), medications, cancer, sarcoidosis, chronic left ventricular failure, and aspiration secondary to pharyngeal dysfunction.

⬛⬛ QuEST: Quickly and Accurate Assess the Patient Using SCHOLAR MAC

QuEST SCHOLAR is an acronym used to assess a patient to determine self-care candidate status and to identify which treatment would be most appropriate. See Chapter 1 for a description of the QuEST SCHOLAR process.

⬛ Does the Patient Have Cough?

- Coughs are described as nonproductive or productive.
    - Nonproductive coughs (dry or "hacking"), which are associated with viral and atypical bacterial infections, GERD, cardiac disease, and some medications, serve no useful physiologic purpose.

- Productive coughs (wet or "chesty") expel secretions from the lower respiratory tract that, if retained, could impair ventilation and the lungs' ability to resist infection. Productive coughs may be effective (secretions easily expelled) or ineffective (secretions present but difficult to expel).

- See Table 1 for signs and symptoms of disorders associated with cough. These should be considered in the patient assessment.

Important SCHOLAR MAC Considerations

- Is the cough nonproductive or productive?

- If the cough is nonproductive, what medications is the patient taking, or has there been a recent change in the medications the patient is taking?
    - Angiotensin-converting enzyme (ACE) inhibitors can cause a dry cough.

- If the cough is productive, what color are the secretions? Is there an odor?
    - Clear secretions typically indicate bronchitis and purulent secretions with bacterial infection.
    - Anaerobic bacterial infections are associated with a distinct malodor.

- What is the duration of the cough?
    - Only acute (<3 weeks) coughs should be treated with nonprescription therapies.

- Does the patient smoke tobacco products?

TABLE 1. Signs and symptoms of disorders associated with cough

Disease	Signs and Symptoms
Acute bronchitis	Purulent sputum; cough that lasts 1–3 weeks; mild dyspnea; mild bronchospasm and wheezing; usually afebrile, although a low-grade fever may be present
Asthma	Wheezing or chest tightness; shortness of breath; coughing predominantly at night; cough in response to specific irritants, such as dust, smoke, or pollen
Chronic bronchitis	Productive cough most days of the month at least 3 months of the year for at least 2 consecutive years
COPD	Persistent, progressive dyspnea; chronic cough (may be intermittent or unproductive); chronic sputum production
GERD	Heartburn, sour taste in mouth, worsening of symptoms in supine position, improvement with acid-lowering drugs
HF	Fatigue, dependent edema, breathlessness
Lower respiratory tract infection	Fever (mild to high); thick, purulent, discolored phlegm; tachypnea, tachycardia
UACS	Mucus drainage from nose; frequent throat clearing
Viral URTI	Sneezing; sore throat; rhinorrhea; low-grade fever

Abbreviations used: HF, heart failure; UACS, upper airway cough syndrome; URTI, upper respiratory tract infection.

▇ Physical Assessment Techniques

■ Observe the patient for signs of chronic medical conditions, such as wheezing (asthma, COPD), productive cough (COPD), barrel chest (COPD), or enlarged lymph nodes (general infection).

■ Obtain vital signs (e.g., temperature, respiratory rate, pulse, and blood pressure).

■ Auscultate chest to detect wheezing, crackles, and rapid or irregular heartbeat.

▇ ▇ QuⒺST: Establish that the patient is an appropriate self-care candidate

Utilize the information collected in the patient assessment with the treatment algorithm and exclusions for self-care to determine if self-care is appropriate.

▇ Exclusions to Self-Care

Review the treatment algorithm and exclusions for self-care provided at the beginning of the chapter. This section highlights key exclusion criteria.

▇ Medications

■ ACE inhibitors—can cause a dry nonproductive cough.

■ Anticholinergics—potential treatment options can have additive anticholinergic effects, resulting in dryness of the eyes and mucous membranes (mouth, nose, vagina).

■ Beta adrenergic blockers—can cause cough in patients with asthma or COPD.

■ Central nervous system (CNS) depressants—potential treatment options can have additive sedation. In addition, this can lead to increased risk for adverse effects and falls.

■ Monoamine oxidase inhibitors (MAOI)—metabolism of potential treatment options can be decreased, leading to adverse effects.

■ See Table 2 for a list of common drug interactions.

▇ Conditions

■ Cough associated with smoking tobacco products should not be suppressed.

TABLE 2. Clinically important drug-drug interactions with nonprescription antitussive agents

Antitussive	Drug/Drug Class	Potential Interaction	Management/ Preventive Measures
Codeine	Alvimopan	Opioid use increases the risk of alvimopan adverse reactions.	Discontinue opioids at least 7 days before initiating alvimopan.
Codeine	CNS depressants, including alcohol, azelastine, doxylamine, droperidol, hydrocodone, orphenadrine, perampanel, sodium oxybate, suvorexant, tapentadol, thalidomide, and zolpidem	CNS depressants enhance the CNS depressant effect of codeine.	Avoid concurrent use if possible.
Codeine	Strong CYP2D6 inhibitors, including abiraterone, fluoxetine, paroxetine, quinidine, and panobinostat	Strong CYP2D6 inhibitors may block the metabolism of codeine to the active metabolites.	Avoid concurrent use if possible.
Codeine	Eluxadoline	Codeine may enhance eluxadoline-associated constipation.	Avoid concurrent use if possible.
Codeine	Mixed agonist/antagonist opioids, including buprenorphine	Mixed agonist/antagonists may reduce the therapeutic effect of codeine.	Avoid concurrent use if possible.
Codeine	Naltrexone	Naltrexone may reduce the therapeutic effect of codeine.	Avoid concurrent use if possible.
Dextromethorphan	Strong CYP2D6 inhibitors, including abiraterone, fluoxetine, paroxetine, quinidine, and panobinostat	Strong CYP2D6 inhibitors may decrease dextromethorphan metabolism, increasing the psychoactive effects of dextromethorphan.	Avoid concurrent use if possible.
Dextromethorphan	Serotonin modulators, including fluoxetine and paroxetine	Serotonin modulators may increase the risk of psychoactive effects of dextromethorphan.	Avoid concurrent use if possible.
Dextromethorphan	MAOIs, including rasagiline, selegiline, isocarboxazid, phenelzine, and tranylcypromine	MAOIs may increase dextro-methorphan-associated sero-tonergic adverse effects.	Avoid concurrent use if possible.

Abbreviations used: CYP, cytochrome P450.

- Cough associated with COPD could be an exacerbation and requires further workup. In addition, COPD could limit medication selection because of drug-disease interactions and adverse effects.

- Narrow-angle glaucoma, acute asthma exacerbation, stenosing peptic ulcer, and symptomatic prostatic hypertrophy are contraindications to use of first-generation (sedating) antihistamines.

■ Special Populations

- Frail older adults may not be appropriate candidates for self-care; all non-prescription medications should be considered for appropriateness, and reduced dosages are generally appropriate.

- Diphenhydramine may cause excitability, especially in children.

■ ■ QuE⑤T: Suggest appropriate self-care strategies

Select the appropriate treatment option based on the previously collected patient data. Various treatment options are discussed along with clinical pearls and pertinent patient considerations for optimal management.

■ Treatment Options

Nonproductive cough treatment of choice is oral antitussives (cough suppressants).

- FDA-approved active ingredients include codeine, dextromethorphan, diphenhydramine, and chlophedianol.

- The American College of Chest Physicians (ACCP) guidelines recommend codeine or dextromethorphan for short-term symptomatic relief of cough associated with acute and chronic bronchitis and postinfectious subacute cough.[2]

- Codeine
    - Codeine is a Schedule V narcotic available without a prescription in certain states.
    - Adverse effects associated with antitussive doses of codeine include nausea, vomiting, sedation, dizziness, and constipation.

- Dextromethorphan
    - Adverse effects with usual doses of dextromethorphan are uncommon but may include drowsiness, nausea or vomiting, stomach discomfort, or constipation.

- First-Generation (Sedating) Antihistamines
    - The ACCP guidelines recommend a combination of a first-generation "sedating" antihistamine with a decongestant to treat the viral infection–induced postnasal drip associated with the common cold that is most likely the cause of the cough.

- Adverse effects associated with diphenhydramine include drowsiness, disturbed coordination, respiratory depression, CNS depression, and anticholinergic effects (e.g., dry eyes, mouth, nose, vagina; blurred vision; urinary hesitancy and retention; constipation; and reflex tachycardia).

- Chlophedianol
    - Chlophedianol is not addressed in the ACCP guidelines.
    - Adverse effects associated with chlophedianol include excitation, hyperirritability, nightmares, hallucinations, hypersensitivity, and urticaria. Dry mouth, vertigo, visual disturbances, nausea, vomiting, and drowsiness have been associated with large doses.

CAUTIONS FOR ORAL ANTITUSSIVES

- Decreased respiratory drive can occur in patients with impaired respiratory reserve (e.g., asthma, COPD) or preexisting respiratory depression; drug addicts, and individuals who take other respiratory depressants or sedatives, including alcohol, should use codeine with caution.
- Additive CNS depression occurs when antitussives are combined with alcohol, antihistamines, narcotics, benzodiazepines, tranquilizers, and psychotropic medications.
- Codeine in combination with promethazine is abused for the sedative effect.
- Dextromethorphan is contraindicated in patients receiving concomitant MAOIs and for 2 weeks after discontinuation because of the risk of serotonergic syndrome.
- Dextromethorphan is frequently abused for euphoric effects. Potential symptoms include mild stimulation, alcohol-like intoxication, dissociative hallucinations, psychosis, and mania.
- Dextromethorphan overdose symptoms include confusion, excitation, nervousness, irritability, restlessness, and drowsiness, as well as severe nausea and vomiting; respiratory depression may occur with very high doses.
- Because of the increased risk of toxicity, diphenhydramine-containing antitussives should not be used with any other diphenhydramine-containing products, including topical products.

- Topical Antitussives
    - Camphor and menthol are the only FDA-approved topical antitussives.
    - Adverse effects include skin, nose, or eye burning, irritation, or both with topical application.

> ### CAUTIONS FOR TOPICAL ANTITUSSIVES
>
> - Camphor and menthol are toxic if ingested.
> - Ointments, creams, and solutions containing camphor or menthol may splatter and cause serious burns if used near an open flame or placed in hot water or in a microwave oven.
> - Ointment formulations of camphor or menthol should not be used in the nostrils, under the nose, by the mouth, on damaged skin, or with tight bandages.

Productive cough treatment of choice is a protussive (expectorant).

- Protussives
  - Guaifenesin is the only FDA-approved expectorant.
  - Guaifenesin is not recommended for any indication in the ACCP guidelines.
    - Data supporting the efficacy of guaifenesin, especially at non-prescription dosages, are limited. Clinical trials show symptom improvement similar to placebo with no significant differences in sputum volume or other properties.[3]
  - Guaifenesin is generally well tolerated. Adverse effects include nausea, vomiting, dizziness, headache, rash, diarrhea, drowsiness, and stomach pain.

> ### CAUTIONS FOR PROTUSSIVES
>
> - No guaifenesin-drug interactions have been reported.
> - Large doses of guaifenesin, either alone or in combination with other agents, have been associated with renal calculi. Do not take more frequently or higher doses than recommended.

- Complementary Therapy
  - Available evidence does not support the use of complementary therapies for treating cough, and some products have potential safety issues.
  - Honey should not be given to children younger than 1 year because of the risk of botulism.

Special Populations

- Pregnancy
  - Codeine should be used during pregnancy only if the potential benefits outweigh the risks. An increased risk of congenital birth defects

exists if codeine is taken during the first trimester of pregnancy. Nonteratogenic concerns include the risk of neonatal respiratory depression if codeine is taken close to the time of delivery and neonatal withdrawal if codeine is used regularly during the pregnancy.

- Dextromethorphan is viewed as probably safe for use during pregnancy.
- Some cough formulations contain alcohol, which is a known teratogen and should be avoided during pregnancy.

- **Breastfeeding**
  - Codeine is excreted in breast milk and is associated with drowsiness in nursing infants.
  - It is not known whether dextromethorphan, chlophedianol, or guaifenesin are excreted in breast milk.
  - Diphenhydramine is excreted in breast milk and may cause unusual excitation and irritability in the infant; it may also decrease the flow of milk.

- **Pediatric Patients**
  - Manufacturers of pediatric cough and cold products have voluntarily revised product labeling to state that the products should not be used in children less than 4 years of age.
  - The efficacy and safety of codeine and dextromethorphan as antitussive drugs in children have not been established.
    - In 2017, the FDA added a contradiction against the use of codeine to treat cough or pain in children younger than 12 years of age and a new warning against the use of codeine in adolescents between 12 and 18 years of age who are obese, have obstructive sleep apnea, or have severe lung disease.
  - Children may experience paradoxical excitation, restlessness, and irritability with diphenhydramine.
  - Ingestion of camphor may be lethal in children.
  - Children typically cannot blow their own noses until 2 years of age; carefully clearing the nasal passageways with a bulb syringe may reduce cough if associated with postnasal drip.

- **Geriatric Patients**
  - Older adults may be more susceptible to the sedating effects of antitussives. The dose should be started at the lower end of the recommended range and titrated as tolerated, with careful monitoring.
  - Older adults are more likely to experience dizziness, excessive sedation, syncope, confusion, and hypotension with diphenhydramine. The 2015 American Geriatrics Society Beers Criteria identify diphenhydramine as potentially inappropriate medication in older adults.

■ ■ QuES▢: Talk with the patient

■ *Patient Education/Counseling*

■ Nonpharmacologic Talking Points

- Nonmedicated lozenges and hard candies may reduce cough by stimulating saliva, thereby decreasing throat irritation.
- Humidifiers increase the amount of moisture in inspired air, which may soothe irritated airways. Cool mist humidifiers and vaporizers are preferred because fewer bacteria grow at the cooler temperatures, and there is less risk of scalding if they are tipped over.
- Less viscous and thus easier-to-expel secretions are formed when the patient is well hydrated. Cautious hydration is recommended for patients with lower respiratory tract infections, heart failure, renal failure, or other medical conditions potentially exacerbated by overhydration.
- Upright positioning and use of nasal bulb syringe are first-line strategies in infants and children who are not eligible for pharmacologic therapy or if cough is associated with postnasal drip.

■ Pharmacologic Talking Points

- Oral Antitussives
  - Cough suppressants are typically used "as needed." Because of the potential for daytime drowsiness, they can be used at night to help suppress cough to allow for sleep.
  - Codeine, dextromethorphan, diphenhydramine, and chlophedianol interact with drugs that cause drowsiness (e.g., narcotics, sedatives, some antihistamines, alcohol).
- Topical Antitussives
  - Slowly dissolve mediated lozenges; do not chew or swallow whole.
  - Medicated lozenges should be used with caution or not at all in young children to avoid the risk of choking.
  - Follow the recommended dosing guidelines; do not overuse.
  - Ointment formulations of camphor or menthol should not be used in the nostrils, under the nose, by the mouth, on damaged skin, or with tight bandages.
- Protussives
  - Staying well hydrated while taking expectorants can help the product to thin secretions.

- Suggest medical referral if any of the following occur:
  - Symptoms worsen while taking nonprescription medications or do not decrease after 1 to 3 weeks of treatment
  - Symptoms develop of a secondary bacterial infection (e.g., thick, colored nasal or respiratory secretions, oral temperature higher than 101.5°F [38.6°C], shortness of breath, chest congestion, wheezing, significant ear pain, rash)

Clinical Pearls

- The underlying cause of the cough must be determined and treated to stop the cough.

- Combinations of antitussives and protussives are potentially counterproductive.

- The AACP guidelines suggest that the anti-inflammatory drug naproxen may reduce viral-associated cough by reducing upper respiratory nerve sensitivity associated with the infection.

- Select single-entity products as much as possible, even if this requires use of two or three products. Treatment should be directed at the most bothersome symptom(s). Only recommend combination products to the patient when all ingredients are indicated for symptom management.

References

1. Tietze K. Cough. In: Krinsky DL, Ferreri SP, Hemstreet BA, Hume AL, Newton GD, Rollins CJ, Tietze KJ, eds. *Handbook of Nonprescription Drugs: An Interactive Approach to Self-Care*. Washington, DC: American Pharmacists Association; 2017:217–230.

2. Irwin RS, Baumann MH, Bolser DC, et al. Diagnosis and management of cough executive summary: ACCP evidence-based clinical practice guidelines. *Chest.* 2006 Jan;129(1 Suppl):1S–23S.

3. Hoffer-Schaefer A, Rozycki HJ, Yopp MA, Rubin BK. Guaifenesin has no effect on sputum volume or sputum properties in adolescents and adults with acute respiratory tract infections. *Respir Care.* 2014 May;59(5):631–636.

DERMATITIS

Nabila Ahmed-Sarwar, PharmD, BCPS, BCACP, CDE, BC-ADM

For complete information on these topics, consult Chapter 33, "Atopic Dermatitis and Dry Skin," written by Kimberley W. Benner; Chapter 35, "Contact Dermatitis," written by Patricia l. Darbishire and Kimberly S. Plake; and Chapter 36, "Diaper Dermatitis and Prickly Heat," written by Katelyn Alexander and Cortney Mospan, published in the *Handbook of Nonprescription Drugs*, 19th Edition.

◼ ◼ Introduction

- A number of dermatologic disorders characterized by erythema and inflammation can be described utilizing the term "dermatitis."

- Differentiating between dermatologic disorders is essential for health care providers, as many patients are either undertreated or self-treat with nonprescription medications.

- Atopic dermatitis (AD) involves inflammatory skin conditions that often are erythematous, edematous, papular, and crusty.

- Erythematous skin irritation that is limited to the area covered by a diaper or prolonged exposed to urine, feces, or both is often associated with diaper dermatitis.

- Skin irritation described as erythema, itching, burning, and stinging that occurs in a limited area following exposure to an irritant or allergen may be a result of contact dermatitis.

ATOPIC DERMATITIS

Self-Care of Atopic Dermatitis

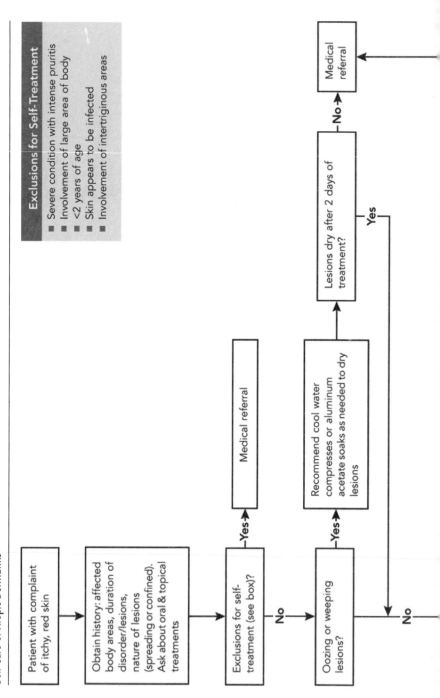

Exclusions for Self-Treatment

- Severe condition with intense pruritis
- Involvement of large area of body
- <2 years of age
- Skin appears to be infected
- Involvement of intertriginous areas

Patient with complaint of itchy, red skin

↓

Obtain history: affected body areas, duration of disorder/lesions, nature of lesions (spreading or confined). Ask about oral & topical treatments

↓

Exclusions for self-treatment (see box)?

— Yes → Medical referral

No ↓

Oozing or weeping lesions?

— Yes → Recommend cool water compresses or aluminum acetate soaks as needed to dry lesions

→ Lesions dry after 2 days of treatment?

— No → Medical referral

Yes ↓

No

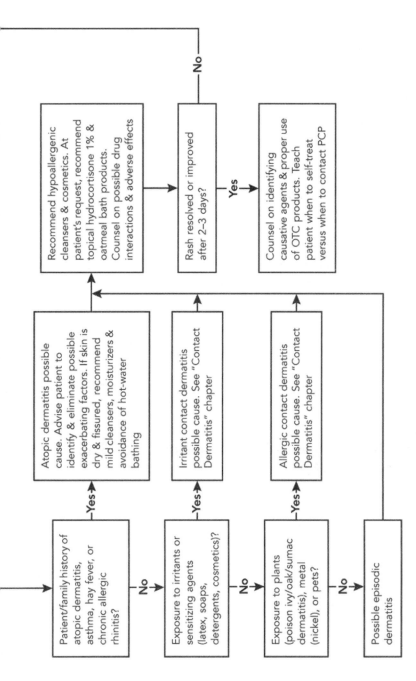

Patient/family history of atopic dermatitis, asthma, hay fever, or chronic allergic rhinitis?

Yes → Atopic dermatitis possible cause. Advise patient to identify & eliminate possible exacerbating factors. If skin is dry & fissured, recommend mild cleansers, moisturizers & avoidance of hot-water bathing

No ↓

Exposure to irritants or sensitizing agents (latex, soaps, detergents, cosmetics)?

Yes → Irritant contact dermatitis possible cause. See "Contact Dermatitis" chapter

No ↓

Exposure to plants (poison ivy/oak/sumac dermatitis), metal (nickel), or pets?

Yes → Allergic contact dermatitis possible cause. See "Contact Dermatitis" chapter

No ↓

Possible episodic dermatitis

Recommend hypoallergenic cleansers & cosmetics. At patient's request, recommend topical hydrocortisone 1% & oatmeal bath products. Counsel on possible drug interactions & adverse effects

↓

Rash resolved or improved after 2–3 days?

No →

Yes ↓

Counsel on identifying causative agents & proper use of OTC products. Teach patient when to self-treat versus when to contact PCP

OTC = over-the-counter; PCP = primary care provider.

■ ■ Overview

- AD, also known as atopic eczema, is an inflammatory skin disorder with unknown etiology that is characterized by cycles of flares and remission.

- Onset is common in infants 2–3 months of age; remission can occur by 2 years of age. It is not uncommon for AD to continue into adulthood.

- There is no cure for AD—symptom management is the primary approach to care. The goals of self-treatment are to stop the itch-scratch cycle, followed by maintenance of skin hydration, trigger avoidance, and prevention of secondary infections.

■ ■ Pathophysiology

- An increase in inflammatory mediators in response to exogenous substances in combination with genetic factors results in red, itchy, and swollen skin.

- Genetic mutations in the epidermis can compromise the skin barrier in AD. The compromised skin barrier increases exposure to allergens and reduces concentrations of lipids and ceramides, negatively affecting the skin's ability to retain moisture.

- The combination of inflammation and dry skin contributes to the pruritus and possibly even infection and pain.

- Symptoms may be aggravated by exposure to high temperatures and low humidity.

■ ■ QuEST: Quickly and Accurate Assess the Patient Using SCHOLAR MAC

QuEST SCHOLAR is an acronym used to assess a patient to determine self-care candidate status and to identify which treatment would be most appropriate. See Chapter 1 for a description of the QuEST SCHOLAR process.

■ Does the Patient Have Atopic Dermatitis?

- The defining characteristic is an itch that becomes a rash.

- Itchy, red skin with papules (small, firm, elevated lesions) or vesicles (fluid- or air-filled sacs) with secretions is typical during the acute phase of AD.
  - Subacute AD often has papules that have been scratched and scaly plaques.

- Chronic AD often has thickened plaques, and prominent markings on the skin are present.
- The location and severity of symptoms are age-dependent.
  - Infants and children initially experience erythema on their cheeks that may progress to the face, neck, forehead, and extremities.
  - Adult symptoms are less severe; plaques can be red, scaly, weeping, or thick and leathery and can be located in the flexural areas of the elbow and knees, neck, forehead, eyes, and hands.
- Exposure to irritants (e.g., fragrances, bleach, smoke) and allergens (e.g., pollen and pets) may worsen symptoms. It is unclear if a relationship between food allergens and symptom exacerbation exists.

Important SCHOLAR MAC Considerations

- Does patient have visible scratch marks?
  - Indicates acute flare of symptoms and possible increase in risk of infection.
- Does patient have lesions that are oozing?
  - Purulent discharge may indicate infection. In the presence of clear discharge, drying the lesions prior to initiating topical therapy will improve drug absorption.
- What percentage of the patient's body is experiencing symptoms?
  - Application of topical steroids over a significant portion of a patient's body surface area is likely to increase systemic absorption.
- Where are the patient's lesions located?
  - The use of ointments should be avoided in areas of skin folds.

Physical Assessment Techniques

- Visually inspect erythematous areas to identify if there is a presence of pustules, vesicles containing exudate or pus, and yellowish crusting of lesions. These may indicate a secondary bacterial or viral infection, which requires assessment by the patient's health care provider.

QuEST: Establish that the patient is an appropriate self-care candidate

Utilize the information collected in the patient assessment with the treatment algorithm and exclusions for self-care to determine if self-care is appropriate.

■ Exclusions to Self-Care

■ Medications

- Existing topical therapies should be stopped during treatment of AD to not affect absorption of treatments for AD. Furthermore, they may be the cause of the AD.
- Emollients containing alcohol, which is often found in gels, foams, and mousses, should be avoided to prevent excessive drying and worsening of symptoms.
- Hydrocortisone products should be used for a limited time during flare-ups.
- Use of ointments in areas where skin rubs together (e.g., skin folds, between fingers, anogenital region) should be avoided because of the risk of skin maceration.

■ Conditions

- Open and cracked skin should be cleansed with mild non-soap cleansers and water and covered to limit exposure to bacteria and viruses. The use of hydrocortisone should be avoided if skin is infected, open, or cracked.
- If more than 10% of body surface area is affected, prescription therapeutic options may be required.

■ Special Populations

- Infants less than 1 year of age have an increased risk of systemic drug absorption because of the smaller body surface area.
- Infants less than 1 year of age will be more sensitive to drying effects of products containing alcohol.

■ ■ QuE⑤T: Suggest appropriate self-care strategies

Select the appropriate treatment option based on previously collected patient data. Various treatment options are discussed along with clinical pearls and pertinent patient considerations for optimal management.

■ Treatment Options

Atopic dermatitis treatment of choice for acute flare-ups is a topical corticosteroid.

- Hydrocortisone
  - Use for acute flare-ups for up to 7 days.
    - Can use on all areas of the body (excluding mucus membranes) for children 2 years of age and older
  - Hydrocortisone should be applied in a thin layer before application of an emollient 1–2 times a day to dry lesions.
  - Ointments effectively penetrate the dermis and are preferred specifically in areas of thick, dry, scaly skin. Evidence supporting ointments over creams is limited; creams may be recommended for patients who do not desire the greasy feel of ointments.
  - Adverse effects are uncommon because of minimal absorption of topical products. The occurrence of skin atrophy is rare with non-prescription concentrations of hydrocortisone. Patients may experience some burning or irritation that is self-limiting.

CAUTIONS FOR TOPICAL CORTICOSTEROIDS

- Avoid ointments if lesions are weeping.
- Continued use may result in reduced response to hydrocortisone. Limiting use to daily only during flare-ups and once weekly dosing or no hydrocortisone during remission phases can help prevent worsening of symptoms.

Atopic dermatitis treatment of choice for dry skin are emollients and moisturizers.

- Moisturizers and Emollients
  - Emollients often contain petrolatum (e.g., Eucerin cream, Lubriderm lotion, and Neutrogena Body Oil).
  - Emollients with ceramides or pseudoceramides (e.g., CeraVe moisturizing cream, Eucerin Professional Repair) assist in preventing moisture loss and contributing to skin repair.
  - Moisturizers and emollients are used in all phases of AD to maintain skin hydration and flexibility.
  - These products should be used in combination with hydrocortisone during acute flare-ups.
  - A variety of dosage formulations are available. Oils may be better suited for hairy areas for better absorption; lotions may be preferred in warmer weather.

▪ Adverse effects are not typically associated with emollients other than potential stains on clothing, bed sheets, etc.

> **CAUTIONS FOR EMOLLIENTS**
> ▪ Avoid emollients with high water content, as they may have a drying effect.
> ▪ Avoid emollients containing fragrances, dyes, and exotic oils to limit the potential for contact irritation.

Other Treatment Considerations

▪ *Itching*, a cardinal symptom of AD, may be caused by several factors, including inflammation and histamine response to trigger exposure.
  ▪ Topical anesthetics (e.g., lidocaine, benzocaine) are not recommended.
  ▪ Topical antihistamines (e.g., diphenhydramine) may provide short-term relief but are not recommended because of their potential to worsen itching.
  ▪ Oral first-generation ("sedating") antihistamines have not been proven effective for itching associated with AD. Use as a sleep aid for patients with difficulty sleeping secondary to itching may be considered.

▪ *Skin infections* can be common because of a compromised skin barrier and introduction of bacteria caused by scratching.
  ▪ Topical antibiotics are not recommended, as they do not appear to improve patient outcomes.
  ▪ Suspected skin infections should be referred to a health care provider for evaluation and treatment.

▪ Complementary Therapy
  ▪ Limited evidence supports the use of topical coconut oil in mild-moderate AD.
  ▪ Probiotic (*Lactobacillus* strains) use in infants was not found to be effective in reducing the presentation of AD symptoms.
  ▪ Phototherapy may be considered a second-line therapy for treatment of acute and chronic AD.

Special Populations

▪ Pregnancy
  ▪ Fetal exposure is unlikely because of minimal systemic absorption. The use of topical steroids and emollients is likely safe in pregnancy.

■ Breastfeeding

- ▪ Limited data exist regarding the expression of topical hydrocortisone in breastmilk. Nursing mothers should avoid utilizing topical products in areas that come in direct contact with the nursing infant to prevent contact irritation.

■ Pediatric Patients

- ▪ Infants have a higher body surface area–to–weight ratio; this increases the proportion of drug absorbed per kilogram. The systemic exposure to topical medications may not be fully metabolized because of their immature hepatic system. Referral to a pediatrician is needed prior to the use of a topical steroid.
- ▪ The use of nonmedicated emollients is safe in pediatric patients.

■ Geriatric Patients

- ▪ Reduced ability to maintain moisture in the skin increases the prevalence of dry skin in older adults, requiring more frequent use of moisturizers throughout the day.
- ▪ Older adults have more fragile skin that may result in increased absorption of the topical corticosteroids.

■ ● QuES◻: Talk with the patient

● *Patient Education/Counseling*

■ Nonpharmacologic Talking Points

- ▪ Avoid common triggers that can irritate skin. Mild non-soap cleansers (e.g., Cetaphil) that are hypoallergenic are preferred. See Table 1 for a list of common triggers associated with AD.
- ▪ Bathe in tepid water for brief periods (3–5 minutes) no more than 3 times a week. Substitute sponge baths when possible.

TABLE 1. Triggers associated with AD

Food allergens (e.g., egg, milk, peanut, soy, wheat, nuts)	Electric blankets
Aeroallergens (e.g., dust mites, cat dander, molds, grass, ragweed, pollen)	Excessive hand or skin washing
Stress	Use of irritating soaps, detergents, and scrubs
Airborne irritants (tobacco smoke, air pollution, traffic exhaust)	Tight-fitting or irritating clothes (wool or synthetics)
Cosmetics, fragrances, and astringents	Dyes and preservatives
Exposure to temperature extremes (heat or cold)	

- Pat dry and apply emollient or moisturizer within 3 minutes of exiting bath to maximize skin hydration.
- Consider wearing cotton gloves or socks on hands at night to limit scratching.
- Cool tap water compresses may be applied to weeping lesions to facilitate drying for 5–20 minutes, 4–6 times a day.

- Pharmacologic Talking Points
  - Hydrocortisone
    - Limit use of hydrocortisone to periods of acute flares:
      - Apply a thin layer and rub into skin thoroughly 2–3 times a day for no longer than 7 days.
    - Wash hands before and after application.
    - Symptom improvement should occur within 24–48 hours of beginning treatment.
    - Avoid contact with mucous membranes.
    - Hydrocortisone should be applied before application of the emollient to ensure proper absorption.
  - Emollients and Moisturizers
    - Apply at minimum 3 times a day to prevent and treat acute flares. More frequent application may be required in areas that are cleansed multiple times a day.
    - Creams, lotions, and oils should be applied liberally.
    - Ointments and butters may be warmed between hands followed by an application of a thin layer massaged into the skin thoroughly.

- Suggest medical referral if any of the following occur:
  - No improvement or worsening of symptoms after 2–3 days of treatment

Clinical Pearls

- Maintaining skin hydration through liberal use of moisturizers and trigger avoidance is essential in the management of AD symptoms.

- Recommend drying oozing or weeping lesions with cool water compresses or aluminum acetate prior to initiating topical therapies.

- Patients with frequent flare-ups may require a "hydrocortisone holiday" or evaluation by a provider to assess for worsening of symptoms.

DIAPER DERMATITIS

Self-Care of Diaper Dermatitis

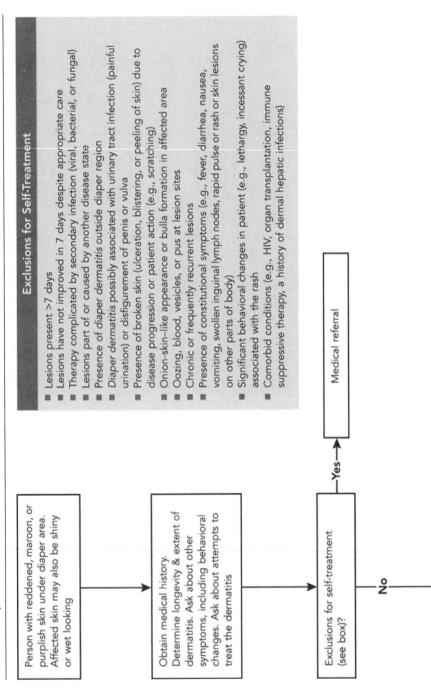

Person with reddened, maroon, or purplish skin under diaper area. Affected skin may also be shiny or wet looking

↓

Obtain medical history. Determine longevity & extent of dermatitis. Ask about other symptoms, including behavioral changes. Ask about attempts to treat the dermatitis

↓

Exclusions for self-treatment (see box)?

— Yes → Medical referral

No

Exclusions for Self-Treatment

- Lesions present >7 days
- Lesions have not improved in 7 days despite appropriate care
- Therapy complicated by secondary infection (viral, bacterial, or fungal)
- Lesions part of or caused by another disease state
- Presence of diaper dermatitis outside diaper region
- Diaper dermatitis possibly associated with urinary tract infection (painful urination) or disfigurement of penis or vulva
- Presence of broken skin (ulceration, blistering, or peeling of skin) due to disease progression or patient action (e.g., scratching)
- Onion-skin–like appearance or bulla formation in affected area
- Oozing, blood, vesicles, or pus at lesion sites
- Chronic or frequently recurrent lesions
- Presence of constitutional symptoms (e.g., fever, diarrhea, nausea, vomiting, swollen inguinal lymph nodes, rapid pulse or rash or skin lesions on other parts of body)
- Significant behavioral changes in patient (e.g., lethargy, incessant crying) associated with the rash
- Comorbid conditions (e.g., HIV, organ transplantation, immune suppressive therapy, a history of dermal hepatic infections)

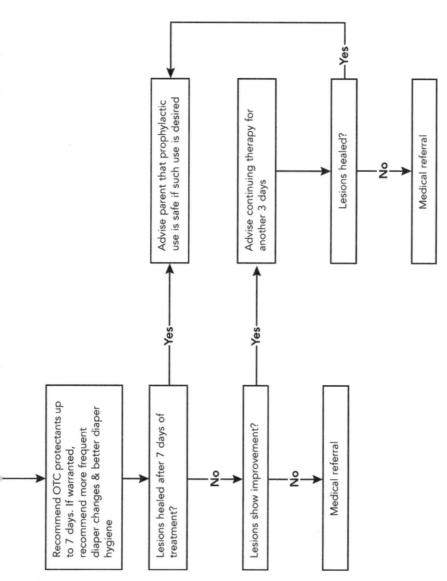

HIV = human immunodeficiency virus; OTC = over-the-counter.

██ Overview

- Diaper dermatitis, commonly known as "diaper rash," involves acute inflammation of the skin of the perineum, buttocks, lower abdomen, and inner thighs.

- Diaper dermatitis is most prevalent in infants less than 2 years of age, yet it can occur in the adult population who experience incontinence. Diaper dermatitis can be prevented by limiting exposure to moisture and feces.

- The optimal treatment approach involves both pharmacological and non-pharmacological measures. The goal of self-treatment is to reduce redness, itching, and discomfort, resolve the rash, prevent secondary infections, and prevent recurrences.

██ Pathophysiology

- The delicate nature of infant perineal skin, exposure to moisture, fecal microbes, and changes in skin pH in combination with the occlusion and friction of a diaper contribute to the development of diaper dermatitis.

- Frequent urination and defecation in conjunction with infrequent diaper changes increases skin moisture. Excessive exposure to moisture obstructs sweat glands, compromising the skin barrier, which increases susceptibility to abrasion and absorption of chemicals and microbes.

- The pH of skin rises secondary to an increase in ammonia levels produced in urine when in contact with fecal bacteria. The change in pH can contribute to skin breakdown.

██ QuEST: Quickly and Accurate Assess the Patient Using SCHOLAR MAC

QuEST SCHOLAR is an acronym used to assess a patient to determine self-care candidate status and to identify which treatment would be most appropriate. See Chapter 1 for a description of the QuEST SCHOLAR process.

▉ Does the Patient Have Diaper Dermatitis?

- Skin patches in the diaper area or accompanying areas that appear red to bright red on children with light skin and may appear maroon or purplish on darker skin.

- Lesions are located in either the groin or perineum areas covered by the diaper. Severe cases can spread outside the diaper area.
  - Infants that lie on their stomach are likely to experience symptoms anterior to their perineum; similarly, infants that lie on their backs may experience symptoms posterior to their perineum.

- Affected skin becomes sensitive, leading to children becoming irritable, fussy, and agitated.

- Onset is in a matter of hours. Skin breakdown transitions quickly from healthy to erythematous.

● Important SCHOLAR MAC Considerations

- Have you noticed a change in the child's activity level or appetite?
  - Lethargy, inconsolable crying, or decreased appetite may indicate systemic infection or possible urinary tract infection.

- Is there skin breakdown?
  - Use of ointments increases the risk of infection. Use of topical skin protectants may prevent healing.

- How often does the child experience diaper dermatitis?
  - Occurrence of more than 4 episodes in 1 month indicates an undiagnosed medical condition if caregivers are utilizing appropriate preventative measures.

● Physical Assessment Techniques

- Utilize open-ended questions to determine the appearance, location, and severity of symptoms.

- Inquire if a rash is present in other areas of the body that are not in the diaper area, as this may indicate a condition other than diaper dermatitis.

- Temperature and heart rate should be monitored in addition to a visual inspection of lymph nodes for swelling if infection is suspected.

■ ■ QuⒺST: Establish that the patient is an appropriate self-care candidate

Utilize the information collected in the patient assessment with the treatment algorithm and exclusions for self-care to determine if self-care is appropriate.

■ Exclusions to Self-Care

Review the treatment algorithm and exclusions for self-care provided at the beginning of the chapter. This section highlights key exclusion criteria.

■ Medications

■ Skin protectants do not interact with other medications but have the potential to occlude other topical medications, increasing the potential for greater systemic absorption.

■ Conditions

■ Diaper dermatitis that occurs outside the areas that are exposed to the wetness should be evaluated by a pediatrician. Diaper dermatitis should be limited to areas covered by the diaper or those that are exposed to mechanical friction (e.g., inner thighs).

■ History of allergies or contact dermatitis may be exacerbated with the use of lanolin.

■ Avoid the use of talc and lipid soluble products (e.g., ointments, zinc oxide, petrolatum) if skin is broken, oozing, or both.

■ Special Populations

■ Older adults may self-treat symptoms of diaper dermatitis, as the systemic absorption of treatment options is minimal.

■ ■ QuE⑤T: Suggest appropriate self-care strategies

Select the appropriate treatment option based on the previously collected patient data. Various treatment options are discussed along with clinical pearls and pertinent patient considerations for optimal management.

■ Treatment Options

Diaper dermatitis treatment of choice is topical skin protectants.

■ Topical Creams, Ointments, Lotions, and Balms
  ■ Use of a combination of FDA-approved skin protectants is acceptable. Commercially available products often are formulated with more than one agent.
    ▫ Table 2 provides FDA-approved skin protectants.

TABLE 2. FDA-approved skin protectants to treat diaper rash

Agent	Concentration (%)
Allantoin	0.5–2
Aluminum hydroxide[a]	0.15–5
Calamine	1–25
Cocoa butter	50–100
Cod liver oil (in combination)	5.0–13.56
Colloidal oatmeal	≤0.007
Dimethicone	1–30
Glycerin[a]	20–45
Hard fat	50–100
Kaolin	4–20
Lanolin	12.5–50
Mineral oil	50–100
Petrolatum	30–100
Topical cornstarch	10–98
White petrolatum	30–100
Zinc carbonate	0.2–2
Zinc oxide	1–25

[a]Consultation with a pediatrician is suggested prior to use in infants.

- Skin protectants may be used prophylactically to prevent recurrent or severe diaper dermatitis.
- Use of petrolatum provides an excellent barrier for the skin against moisture.
- Zinc oxide is available in ointment and creamlike washable formulations. In comparison to washable formulations, ointments require soap and water to remove but provide a better protective layer against moisture.
- Lanolin has bacteriostatic properties. Use should be carefully evaluated because of the potential to cause contact dermatitis.
- Calamine has absorptive, antiseptic, and antipruritic properties.
- Mineral oil is most often used in small quantities as an inactive ingredient. The buildup of mineral oil in pores can lead to folliculitis.
- Dimethicone, a silicone-based oil, is often used in combination with other products to provide a barrier and possible anti-inflammatory effects.
- There are no common adverse effects from the use of skin protectants because of their lack of systemic absorption.

> **CAUTIONS FOR TOPICAL CREAMS, OINTMENTS, LOTIONS, AND BALMS**
> - The use of non-FDA-approved ingredients found in diaper dermatitis products (e.g., castor oil, beeswax, chamomile, honey, jojoba) should be avoided.
> - Monitor for worsening of symptoms with lanolin use, indicating contact sensitization.

- Topical Loose Powders
  - These products (e.g., cornstarch, talc) provide benefit by reducing moisture and friction, but they should generally be avoided because of inhalation risk.
  - Cornstarch has absorptive properties to help reduce moisture.
  - Talc serves as a lubricant to minimize mechanical irritation.

> **CAUTIONS FOR TOPICAL CORNSTARCH**
> - Inhalation of loose powders is associated with severe respiratory disease. If possible, an alternative agent should be used to limit this risk.
> - Talc should not be applied to broken or oozing skin, as it can cause infection or slow healing.

Other Treatment Considerations

- *Skin irritation* that clinically presents as erythema is a cardinal symptom of diaper dermatitis. The use of hydrocortisone is not recommended to relieve the irritation, as it increases the risk of secondary infections because of the suppression of immune response.
- *Pain* that may clinically present as irritability, fussiness, and agitation should be managed by minimizing mechanical friction. The use of topical analgesics is not recommended, as children are unable to communicate pain perception. Topical analgesics may damage the skin and slow the skin healing process.

- Complementary Therapy
  - Insufficient evidence exists in regard to complementary therapies; unknown absorption rates may pose a risk to children.
  - Limited studies have shown honey, beeswax, and olive oil to be effective for diaper dermatitis in adults. Additional studies are needed prior to recommending these agents.

◼ *Special Populations*

- ▪ Pediatric Patients
  - ▫ The use of topical agents is safe in pediatric patients.
- ▪ Geriatric Patients
  - ▫ The use of topical agents is safe in older adults.

◼ ◼ QuES❶: Talk with the patient

◼ *Patient Education/Counseling*

- ▪ Nonpharmacologic Talking Points
  - ▫ Reduce contact of skin with diaper by implementing even a brief "diaper holiday," exposing the affected skin to air to limit exposure to moisture and promote healing.
  - ▫ Change diapers more frequently, at a minimum, every 2 hours in newborns and every 3–4 hours in older infants.
    - ▫ Diapers should be changed immediately following a bowel movement to minimize exposure to fecal bacteria.
    - ▫ Do not use any part of the soiled diaper to wipe the child.
  - ▫ Cleanse the area by gently patting the skin, limiting cleansing to occasions when stool is present.
    - ▫ Utilizing a baby wipe formulated for sensitive skin or careful rinsing of skin with warm water followed by non-friction drying reduces mechanical irritation.
    - ▫ Allow thorough air drying prior to rediapering.
  - ▫ Use of dye-free disposable diapers is preferred for their ability to absorb moisture better than cloth diapers, preventing mixing of urine and feces.
    - ▫ If cloth diapers are used, avoid covering with plastic or rubber pants, and wash in mild detergent.
- ▪ Pharmacologic Talking Points
  - ▪ Topical Creams, Ointments, Lotions, Balms
    - ▫ Wash hands thoroughly prior to and after applying the topical product.
    - ▫ Prior to applying the skin protectant, gently cleanse the diaper area with plain water and allow to thoroughly dry.

- Overuse of an agent is not of concern; remaining protectant from the previous diaper change does not need to be removed.
    - Mineral oil should be washed off with every diaper change to avoid folliculitis.
- Frequent use of generous amounts with every diaper change is recommended, focusing on erythematous areas.
- Avoid applying other topical formulations over ointment formulations, as the ointments limit their ability to be absorbed.
- Improvement commonly occurs within 24 hours of implementing pharmacologic and nonpharmacologic therapies.
  - Topical Powders
    - To limit the risk of inhalation, caregivers should pour powder into their hands away from the child and gently pat it onto the affected area.

- Suggest medical referral if any of the following occur:
  - No sign of improvement or resolution after seven days of treatment

Clinical Pearls

- The mnemonic "ABCDE" (air, barrier, cleansing, diaper, and education) may be used to remember the treatment modalities used to treat diaper dermatitis.

- The "more is better" approach should be encouraged when applying skin protectants to provide an adequate barrier to the skin.

- Clinical evidence is lacking to support the use of extemporaneous compounded products, such as aluminum hydroxide suspension (Maalox) combined with Aquaphor or the combination of aluminum acetate, petrolatum, and zinc oxide.

CONTACT DERMATITIS

Self-Care of Contact Dermatitis

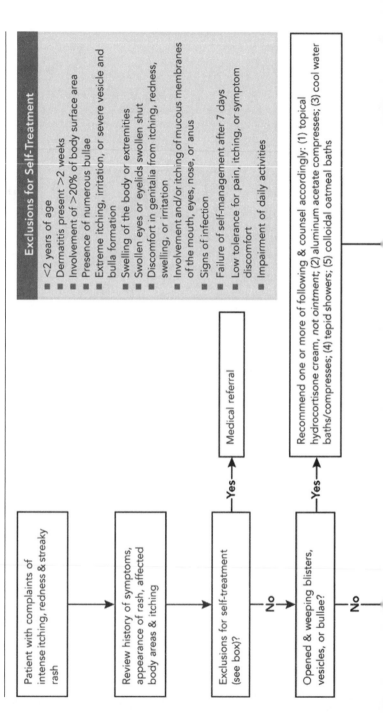

Patient with complaints of intense itching, redness & streaky rash

↓

Review history of symptoms, appearance of rash, affected body areas & itching

↓

Exclusions for self-treatment (see box)? —Yes→ Medical referral

↓ No

Opened & weeping blisters, vesicles, or bullae? —Yes→ Recommend one or more of following & counsel accordingly: (1) topical hydrocortisone cream, *not ointment*; (2) aluminum acetate compresses; (3) cool water baths/compresses; (4) tepid showers; (5) colloidal oatmeal baths

↓ No

Exclusions for Self-Treatment

- <2 years of age
- Dermatitis present >2 weeks
- Involvement of >20% of body surface area
- Presence of numerous bullae
- Extreme itching, irritation, or severe vesicle and bulla formation
- Swelling of the body or extremities
- Swollen eyes or eyelids swollen shut
- Discomfort in genitalia from itching, redness, swelling, or irritation
- Involvement and/or itching of mucous membranes of the mouth, eyes, nose, or anus
- Signs of infection
- Failure of self-management after 7 days
- Low tolerance for pain, itching, or symptom discomfort
- Impairment of daily activities

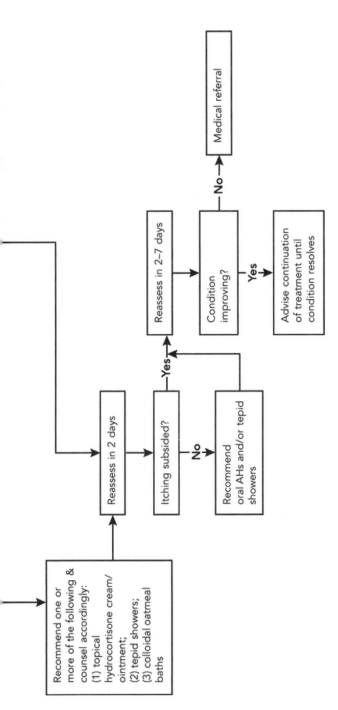

AH = antihistamine.

■ ■ Overview

■ Contact dermatitis can be classified as either irritant contact dermatitis (ICD) or allergic contact dermatitis (ACD).

■ The presence of existing skin conditions pre-exposes a patient to experience profound dermatitis symptoms because of the increased permeability of the dermis.

■ As frequency of exposure and concentration of an irritant increase, the severity of dermatitis also increases.

■ The goals of self-treatment are to remove the irritant or allergen, prevent further contact, relieve inflammation and irritation, and prevent secondary infections.

   ■ Goals for self-treatment of ACD include relief from pruritus and clearing the skin of any crust that forms or scaling that occurs as the vesicles heal.

■ ■ Pathophysiology

■ Irritant Contact Dermatitis (ICD)

   ■ The primary cause of ICD is an inflammatory response caused by exposure to an irritant substance that results in destruction of the epidermis.

   ■ Following exposure to an irritant, the skin's barrier is disrupted, and a release of inflammatory mediators occurs.

      □ Conditions leading to enhanced permeability of the dermis, such as AD, warm temperatures, and high humidity, may predispose a patient to a more profound response to irritant exposure.

   ■ Repeated exposure to mild irritants (e.g., detergents, soaps, dyes) is likely to result in dermatitis in contrast to chemical irritants that result in immediate reactions upon first exposure.

   ■ Individuals who wash their hands, handle food, have repeated contact with irritants, or combinations thereof are more likely to develop ICD.

■ Allergic Contact Dermatitis

   ■ The primary cause of ACD is an immunologic reaction of the skin in response to allergen exposure.

   ■ Antigen exposure results in a hypersensitivity reaction, resulting in dermatitis that can be delayed with first response. Repeated exposure to an antigen results in a quicker immune response, resulting in dermatitis.

- Urushiol-Induced ACD
  - This is an immunologic reaction caused by exposure to urushiol.
    - Urushiol is the antigenic component found in *Toxicodendron* plants (e.g., poison ivy, poison oak, poison sumac).
    - The response to urushiol exposure can begin within 10 minutes of coming in contact with skin.
  - Once urushiol has entered the skin and attached to tissue proteins, the antigenic process begins.
  - Immediate washing and meticulous cleansing under fingernails, clipping of fingernails, or both can help minimize reaction and prevent further spreading of the irritant.
  - Sensitivity to urushiol has been reported in toddlers but is more pronounced in adults. Older adults may not be as sensitive to urushiol exposure, but the resulting dermatitis may delay healing.

Preventative Measures

- Reducing exposure to irritants and allergens is the foundation of preventing ICD and ACD.

- Use protective clothing and gloves when working with irritants or while outside and exposed to vegetation. Urushiol may be transferred from hands or inanimate objects to other parts of the body. It remains active in dead or dried plants or on contaminated objects for several years. Pets are often the cause of transfer to people.

- Immediately wash any exposed surfaces or items to limit the spread of and exposure to urushiol.

- The use of barrier products (e.g., bentonite, kaolin, silicone products) provides limited protection against urushiol exposure.

QuEST: Quickly and Accurate Assess the Patient Using SCHOLAR MAC

QuEST SCHOLAR is an acronym used to assess a patient to determine self-care candidate status and to identify which treatment would be most appropriate. See Chapter 1 for a description of the QuEST SCHOLAR process.

● Does the Patient Have Contact Dermatitis?

- Contact dermatitis is characterized by inflammation, erythema, itching, burning, and stinging that is limited to the area exposed to the irritant or allergen.

- See Table 3 for factors that distinguish between ICD and ACD.

● Does the Patient Have Irritant Contact Dermatitis?

- Characteristics of ICD include stinging and burning early after exposure.

- Exposure to detergents, chemicals, solvents, and salts is more common in ICD.

- Symptoms do not appear immediately after exposure.

- ICD is localized to areas exposed to irritants (e.g., hands and face).

● Does the Patient Have Allergic Contact Dermatitis?

- The presence of vesicles and papules (i.e., rash) is unique to ACD and is not seen in ICD.

TABLE 3. Differentiation of ICD and ACD

Symptom or Characteristic	ICD	ACD
Itching	Yes, later	Yes, early
Stinging, burning	Early	Late or not at all
Erythema	Yes	Yes
Vesicles, bullae	Rarely or no	Yes
Papules	Rarely or no	Yes
Dermal edema	Yes	Yes
Time to reaction (rash) after exposure	Dependent on irritant	Dependent on antigen
Appearance of symptoms in relation to exposures	Initial or repetitive exposures	Delayed for first exposure; in subsequent exposures, varies based on antigen and sensitivity
Causative substances	Water, urine, flour, detergents, hand sanitizers, soap, alkalis, acids, solvents, salts, surfactants, oxidizers	*Toxicodendron* plants, fragrances, nickel, latex, benzocaine, neomycin, leather
Substance concentration at exposure	Important	Less important
Mechanism of reaction	Direct tissue damage	Immunologic reaction
Common location	Hands, wrist, forearms, diaper area	Anywhere on body that comes in contact with antigen
Presentation	No clear margins	Clear margins based on contact of offending substance

- Exposure to *Toxicodendron* plants, fragrances, latex, and medication are common causes of ACD.

- Symptoms do not appear immediately after exposure; the first exposure may produce a mild response, and repeated exposures may result in more intense symptoms.

- Symptoms of ACD can occur anywhere the antigen comes in contact with the body.

Important SCHOLAR MAC Considerations

- Has the patient recently been exposed to any new products that contain irritants (e.g., new laundry detergent, new soap)?
  - Products with high concentrations of irritants may require multiple products to relieve itching and moisturize skin to prevent breakdown.
  - Potential sources of dermatitis should be identified and removed.

- Has the patient recently been outside where they may have encountered poison ivy or poison oak?
  - Emphasize immediate cleansing prior to initiating topical therapies to prevent repeated exposure of urushiol.

- Does the patient have any existing dermatological conditions?
  - Patients may experience more severe reactions and may require multiple products to relieve itching and require moisturizing of skin to prevent breakdown.

- Does the patient have an immunocompromising condition?
  - Immunocompromising conditions (e.g., corticosteroid use, HIV, immunosuppressant use, cancer, and uncontrolled diabetes) may cause delayed wound healing and risk secondary infections. These patients should be carefully managed during follow-up.

Physical Assessment Techniques

- Visually inspect erythematous areas to identify if there are vesicles containing exudate or pus present.

- Oozing or weeping vesicles with clear fluid are common in ACD and can develop a crust; however, yellowish crusting may indicate a secondary infection that needs to be evaluated by a health care provider.

■■ Qu⬛ST: Establish that the patient is an appropriate self-care candidate

Utilize the information collected in the patient assessment with the treatment algorithm and exclusions for self-care to determine if self-care is appropriate.

■ Exclusions to Self-Care

■ Medications

= Oral corticosteroids—colloidal oatmeal may be preferred for relief of itching over topical hydrocortisone, as it is unlikely to provide additional relief when taken with oral steroids.

= Other topical medications—discontinue use on affected area until symptoms are resolved. Application of oil-based topical products or use of occlusive dressings over topical medications may increase systemic absorption and risk of adverse effects.

■ Conditions

= Presence of dermatitis for more than 2 weeks may indicate the presence of an undiagnosed immunosuppressive condition, as most cases self-resolve in 10–21 days.

= Lesions that cover a large portion of the body (~>20% of body surface area) likely require systemic therapy, as application of topical agents over a large surface area becomes difficult, and there is an increased risk of systemic absorption of topical medication.

= Presence of numerous bullae, extreme itching, irritation, or severe vesicles when covered by ointments may prevent proper draining and drying of lesions and increase the risk of infection.

= Application of topical products to the genitalia or mucous membranes (e.g., mouth, nose, eyes) may lead to systemic absorption and increase the risk of adverse effects. Treatment with nonsterile topical products may increase the risk of infection.

■ Special Populations

= Children less than 2 years of age may have an increased risk of drug absorption.

▫ The use of hydrocortisone should be avoided without pediatrician evaluation.

▫ The use of nonmedicated skin protectants, colloidal oatmeal, or mild soap cleansers is safe.

- Older adults may not be able to mount a sufficient immune response for self-healing; nonprescription therapies are focused on symptom management.

◼ ◼ QuE◼T: Suggest appropriate self-care strategies

Select the appropriate treatment option based on previously collected patient data. Various treatment options are discussed along with clinical pearls and pertinent patient considerations for optimal management.

◼ Treatment Options

*Irritant contact dermatitis **skin protection*** treatment of choice is emollients.

- ◼ Emollients
  - Emollients often contain petrolatum (e.g., Eucerin cream, Lubriderm lotion, and Neutrogena Body Oil).
  - Emollients with ceramides or pseudoceramides (e.g., CeraVe moisturizing cream, Eucerin Professional Repair) assist in preventing moisture loss and contributing to skin repair.
  - A variety of dosage formulations are available. Oils may be better suited for hairy areas for better absorption; because of the occlusive nature of ointments, lotions may be preferred in warmer weather.
  - Adverse effects are not typically associated with emollients other than potential stains on clothing, bed sheets, etc.

> **CAUTIONS FOR EMOLLIENTS**
> - Avoid emollients with high water content, as they may have a drying effect.
> - Avoid emollients containing fragrances, dyes, and exotic oils.

*Irritant contact dermatitis **itching*** treatment of choice is colloidal oatmeal

- ◼ Colloidal Oatmeal
  - Bathing in colloidal oatmeal helps relieve itching and cleanses the affected area.
  - Oatmeal baths consist of 1 packet or 1 cup of milled oatmeal mixed thoroughly in tepid bath water. Soaking for 15–20 minutes twice a day followed by gently patting the skin dry helps relieve symptoms.
  - There are no known adverse effects associated with colloidal oatmeal use.

> **CAUTIONS FOR COLLOIDAL OATMEAL**
> - Oatmeal baths can cause the bathtub to become slippery. Caution should be used when entering and exiting to prevent falls.
> - Clogged bathtub drains may occur; use of a drain strainer can help prevent this.

- Hydrocortisone
  - Hydrocortisone is controversial for ICD; the medication does not address the cause but may reduce inflammation and itching.
  - Hydrocortisone should be applied in a thin layer before application of any emollient 1–2 times a day to dry lesions. Avoid applying hydrocortisone to oozing lesions.
  - Evidence supporting ointments over creams is limited; creams may be recommended for patients that do not desire the greasy feel of ointments.
  - The risk of systemic adverse effects is very low because of minimal systemic absorption of topical products. The occurrence of skin atrophy is rare with nonprescription concentrations of hydrocortisone.

Allergic contact dermatitis cleansing treatment of choice is antigen cleansers or mild soaps.

- Antigen Cleansers
  - Washing within 30 minutes of urushiol contact may minimize the antigenic process. Immediate washing is preferred.
  - Available nonprescription products may not be more efficacious and are costlier than using mild soap (e.g., Cetaphil, Dove) and water.
  - Cleansers intended to prevent rash and itching (e.g., Tecnu Original Outdoor Skin Cleanser, Tecnu Extreme Medicated Poison Ivy Scrub, Zanfel) may be used to remove urushiol even after a rash has developed and may provide relief from pain and itching. Other products are intended to prevent rash and itching.
  - There are no know severe adverse effects; minor skin irritation may occur and is self-limiting.

> **CAUTIONS FOR ANTIGEN CLEANSERS**
> - To avoid damaging the skin, avoid vigorous scrubbing of the skin and harsh cleansers (e.g., hand sanitizers, harsh soap, bleach).

Allergic contact dermatitis symptom relief treatment of choice is topical cortico-steroids.

- Hydrocortisone
    - Hydrocortisone relieves itching and inflammation; nonprescription concentrations may not treat the rash effectively.
    - Products may be applied up to 3–4 times a day as initial therapy.
    - Ointments effectively penetrate the dermis and are preferred specifically in areas of thick, dry, scaly skin. Creams assist in drying lesions that may be oozing.
    - The risk of systemic adverse effects is very low because of minimal systemic absorption of topical products. The occurrence of skin atrophy is rare with nonprescription concentrations of hydrocortisone. Patients may experience some burning or irritation that is self-limiting.

> **CAUTIONS FOR TOPICAL CORTICOSTEROIDS**
>
> - Topical corticosteroids are not safe for application over the eyelids.
> - Systemic absorption can occur with prolonged use, with occlusive dressings, with large surface areas, or when skin is broken. Patients should be warned of these symptoms and instructed to watch for them or how to minimize them.

Allergic contact dermatitis weeping lesions treatment of choice is astringents.

- Topical Astringents
    - Astringents cool and dry the skin, helping to reduce edema, exudation, and inflammation.
    - Common astringents may be prepared by the patient at home:
        - Burow's solution (e.g., Domeboro)
        - Isotonic saline solution (1 teaspoon salt in 2 cups of water)
        - Diluted white vinegar (¼ cup in 1 pint of water)
        - Baking soda may be mixed with water to form a solution or paste.
    - A compress soaked in astringent may be applied to the affected area for 20–30 minutes, 4–6 times a day to help soften crusted lesions for removal and can relieve itching.
    - There are no known severe adverse effects; mild irritation may occur that is self-limiting.

> **CAUTIONS FOR ASTRINGENTS**
>
> - Prepare a new solution for each application.

◼ Other Treatment Considerations

■ *Topical ointments and creams* containing anesthetics (e.g., benzocaine), antihistamines (e.g., diphenhydramine), or antibiotics (e.g., neomycin) should not be using for itching related to ACD because of the sensitization risk.

■ *First-generation ("sedating") oral antihistamines* can be used for patients who require nighttime sedation. Use should be avoided in patients sensitive to anticholinergic adverse effects (e.g., benign prostatic hyperplasia, glaucoma) or at risk for falls (e.g., elderly, presence of vertigo).

◼ Special Populations

■ Pregnancy
  ▪ Systemic absorption of topical agents for the treatment of contact dermatitis is minimal; fetal exposure is unlikely.
  ▪ These should not be used for long periods or over extensive areas of the body to prevent systemic absorption.

■ Breastfeeding
  ▪ Limited data exist regarding the expression of topical agents in breastmilk. Lack of systemic absorption supports the use of these agents in breastfeeding mothers.

■ Pediatric Patients
  ▪ The use of topical agents (e.g., emollients, barrier creams, topical corticosteroids) for the treatment of contact dermatitis is safe in pediatric patients 2 years of age and older.

■ Geriatric Patients
  ▪ Priority should be given to reduction in itching because of the increased risk of skin breakdown from scratching.
  ▪ The use of topical agents is safe in older adults.
  ▪ Caution should be used in recommending the use of oral first-generation (sedating) antihistamines for itching because of the risk of sedation.

◼ ◼ QuES⬛: Talk with the patient

◼ Patient Education/Counseling

■ Nonpharmacologic Talking Points
  ▪ Reduce or avoid contact with the irritant or antigen to begin the skin healing process.

- Cold or tepid showers with mild cleansers may relieve itching. Avoid hot showers, as they can further injure the skin and exacerbate itching.
- Maintaining short fingernails that are smooth and clean is important to remove trapped irritants and avoid introduction of bacteria when scratching pruritic areas.

- Pharmacologic Talking Points
  - Wash hands thoroughly prior to and after application of topical agents. Avoid contact with mucous membranes.
  - Hydrocortisone should be applied prior to application of the emollient to ensure proper absorption.
  - Emollients may be used as frequently and applied as liberally as necessary to relieve symptoms.
  - Astringent use should be limited to areas with vesicles, bullae, and weeping lesions.
  - Itching and rash should improve within 5–7 days of self-treatment. Symptoms associated with ACD may take up to three weeks to resolve, but treatment with nonprescription products is not recommended beyond 7 days.

- Suggest medical referral if any of the following occur:
  - If symptoms have not improved or have worsened after 7 days of treatment
  - If the rash covers a large surface area (>20% body surface area) or has increased in size
  - If rash has spread to the eyes, genitals, or face
  - Evidence of systemic involvement (e.g., joint swelling) or secondary infection

Clinical Pearls

- Surfactants (e.g., Dial Ultra dishwashing soap), and oil-removing compounds (e.g., Goop) are just as effective as pharmacological cleansers to protect against poison ivy rash when used to cleanse skin exposed to urushiol.

- Colloidal oatmeal and calamine lotion may be used for symptoms associated with ACD; use should be avoided in the presence of oozing lesions. Appearance of a pink film on the skin is common with calamine use.

- Use of hypoallergenic cleansers, creams, and cosmetics are preferred to reduce the risk of ACD.

● ● References

1. Benner KW. Dermatitis and Dry Skin. In: Krinsky DL, Ferreri SP, Hemstreet BA, Hume AL, Newton GD, Rollins CJ, Tietze KJ, eds. *Handbook of Nonprescription Drugs: An Interactive Approach to Self-Care*. Washington, DC: American Pharmacists Association; 2017:653–666.

2. Alexander K, Mospan C. Diaper Dermatitis and Prickly Heat. In: Krinsky DL, Ferreri SP, Hemstreet BA, Hume AL, Newton GD, Rollins CJ, Tietze KJ, eds. *Handbook of Nonprescription Drugs: An Interactive Approach to Self-Care*. Washington, DC: American Pharmacists Association; 2017:695–708.

3. Darbishire PL, Plake KS. Contact Dermatitis. In: Krinsky DL, Ferreri SP, Hemstreet BA, Hume AL, Newton GD, Rollins CJ, Tietze KJ, eds. *Handbook of Nonprescription Drugs: An Interactive Approach to Self-Care*. Washington, DC: American Pharmacists Association; 2017:681–694.

DIARRHEA

Erin N. Adams, PharmD, BCACP

For complete information about this topic, consult Chapter 16, "Diarrhea," written by Paul C. Walker and published in the *Handbook of Nonprescription Drugs*, 19th Edition.[1]

Self-Care of Acute Diarrhea in Children 6 Months to 5 Years

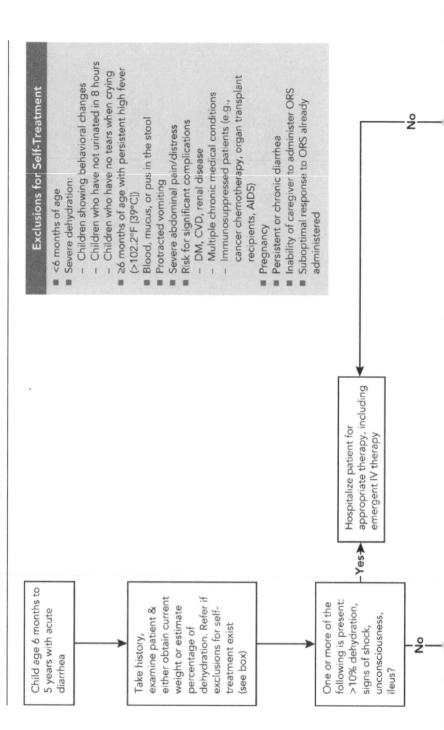

Child age 6 months to 5 years with acute diarrhea

Take history, examine patient & either obtain current weight or estimate percentage of dehydration. Refer if exclusions for self-treatment exist (see box)

One or more of the following is present: >10% dehydration, signs of shock, unconsciousness, ileus?

Yes → Hospitalize patient for appropriate therapy, including emergent IV therapy

No

Exclusions for Self-Treatment

- <6 months of age
- Severe dehydration:
  - Children showing behavioral changes
  - Children who have not urinated in 8 hours
  - Children who have no tears when crying
- ≥6 months of age with persistent high fever (>102.2°F [39°C])
- Blood, mucus, or pus in the stool
- Protracted vomiting
- Severe abdominal pain/distress
- Risk for significant complications
  - DM, CVD, renal disease
  - Multiple chronic medical conditions
  - Immunosuppressed patients (e.g., cancer chemotherapy, organ transplant recipients, AIDS)
- Pregnancy
- Persistent or chronic diarrhea
- Inability of caregiver to administer ORS
- Suboptimal response to ORS already administered

No

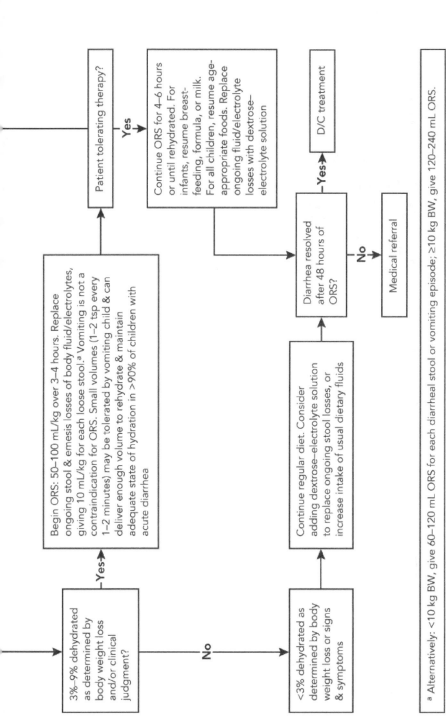

Patient tolerating therapy?

Yes

Continue ORS for 4–6 hours or until rehydrated. For infants, resume breast-feeding, formula, or milk. For all children, resume age-appropriate foods. Replace ongoing fluid/electrolyte losses with dextrose–electrolyte solution

Begin ORS: 50–100 mL/kg over 3–4 hours. Replace ongoing stool & emesis losses of body fluid/electrolytes, giving 10 mL/kg for each loose stool.[a] Vomiting is not a contraindication for ORS. Small volumes (1–2 tsp every 1–2 minutes) may be tolerated by vomiting child & can deliver enough volume to rehydrate & maintain adequate state of hydration in >90% of children with acute diarrhea

3%–9% dehydrated as determined by body weight loss and/or clinical judgment?

Yes

No

D/C treatment

Diarrhea resolved after 48 hours of ORS?

Yes

No

Medical referral

Continue regular diet. Consider adding dextrose–electrolyte solution to replace ongoing stool losses, or increase intake of usual dietary fluids

<3% dehydrated as determined by body weight loss or signs & symptoms

[a] Alternatively: <10 kg BW, give 60–120 mL ORS for each diarrheal stool or vomiting episode; ≥10 kg BW, give 120–240 mL ORS.

AIDS = acquired immunodeficiency syndrome; BW = body weight; CVD = cardiovascular disease; D/C = discontinue; DM = diabetes mellitus; IV = intravenous; ORS = oral rehydration solution.

Self-Care of Acute Diarrhea in Children Older Than 5 Years, Adolescents, and Adults

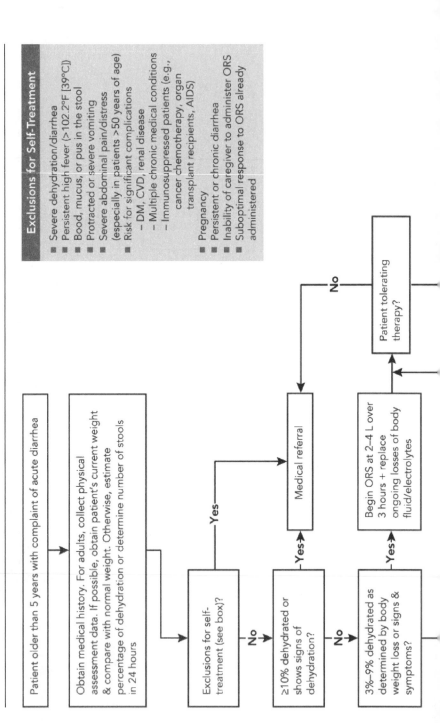

Exclusions for Self-Treatment

- Severe dehydration/diarrhea
- Persistent high fever (>102.2°F [39°C])
- Bood, mucus, or pus in the stool
- Protracted or severe vomiting
- Severe abdominal pain/distress (especially in patients >50 years of age)
- Risk for significant complications
  - DM, CVD, renal disease
  - Multiple chronic medical conditions
  - Immunosuppressed patients (e.g., cancer chemotherapy, organ transplant recipients, AIDS)
- Pregnancy
- Persistent or chronic diarrhea
- Inability of caregiver to administer ORS
- Suboptimal response to ORS already administered

Patient older than 5 years with complaint of acute diarrhea

Obtain medical history. For adults, collect physical assessment data. If possible, obtain patient's current weight & compare with normal weight. Otherwise, estimate percentage of dehydration or determine number of stools in 24 hours

Exclusions for self-treatment (see box)? — Yes → Medical referral

No ↓

≥10% dehydrated or shows signs of dehydration? — Yes →

No ↓

3%–9% dehydrated as determined by body weight loss or signs & symptoms? — Yes → Begin ORS at 2–4 L over 3 hours + replace ongoing losses of body fluid/electrolytes

Patient tolerating therapy?

No →

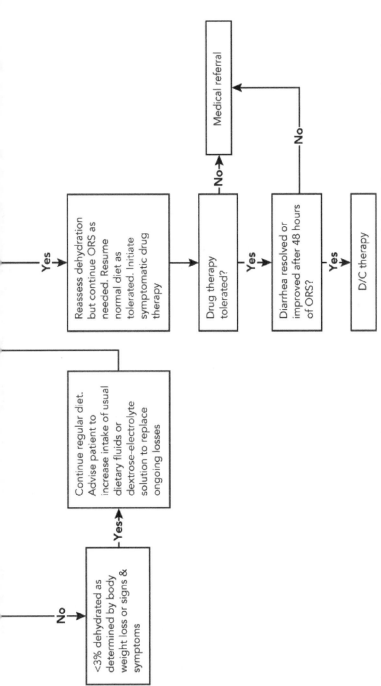

AIDS = acquired immunodeficiency syndrome; CVD = cardiovascular disease; D/C = discontinue; DM = diabetes mellitus; ORS = oral rehydration solution.

■ ■ Overview

- Bowel habits and frequency vary. Diarrhea is characterized as having more than 3 bowel movements per day with an increase in stool frequency, liquidity, or weight.

- The goals of self-treatment are to prevent and correct fluid and electrolyte loss or acid-base disturbances, control symptoms, identify and treat the cause, and prevent acute morbidity and mortality.

■ ■ Pathophysiology

- Diarrhea can be caused by a variety of organisms, including viruses, bacteria, or protozoa.
    - Viral gastroenteritis is most often transmitted by contaminated water or food but can also be transmitted from person to person and through contact with contaminated environmental surfaces.
    - Most cases of bacterial gastroenteritis result from foodborne transmission.
    - Protozoal diarrhea is not appropriate for self-care treatment.

- Diarrhea may be provoked from a food intolerance, a food allergy, or ingestion of foods that are overly fatty, spicy, or contain a high amount of dietary fiber or many seeds.

- Conditions and medications (e.g., irritable bowel syndrome, antibiotics) may induce diarrhea.

■ *Preventative Measures*

- Isolating the individual with diarrhea, washing hands, and using sterile techniques are basic preventive measures that reduce the risk of transmission to other patients and their caregivers.

- Strict food handling, sanitation, and other hygienic practices help control transmission of bacteria as well as other infectious agents.

■ ■ QuEST: Quickly and Accurate Assess the Patient Using SCHOLAR MAC

QuEST SCHOLAR is an acronym used to assess a patient to determine self-care candidate status and to identify which treatment would be most appropriate. See Chapter 1 for a description of the QuEST SCHOLAR process.

● *Does the Patient Have Acute Diarrhea?*

■ Patient should report an increase in stool frequency (e.g., having more than 3 bowel movements per day), liquidity, or weight.

■ Additional symptoms can include nausea, vomiting, and fever.

■ Fluid and electrolyte imbalance leading to dehydration is the major complication of diarrheal illness. See Table 1 for signs and symptoms of dehydration.

● *Important SCHOLAR MAC Considerations*

■ What are the characteristics of the patient's bowel movements?
  ▪ Stool characteristics give valuable information about the diarrhea's pathophysiology.
    ▫ Undigested food particles suggest disease of the small intestine.
    ▫ Black, tarry stools may indicate upper gastrointestinal (GI) bleeding.
    ▫ Red stools suggest lower bowel or hemorrhoid bleeding. This can also result from ingestion of red food (e.g., beets) or medications (e.g., rifampin).
    ▫ Yellowish stools suggest bilirubin and liver disease.
    ▫ Whitish tint to the stool suggests fat malabsorption disease.
    ▫ Many small-volume stools suggest a colonic disorder.

■ How long has the patient been experiencing diarrhea?
  ▪ Diarrhea lasting less than 14 days is generally self-limiting and treatable with self-care measures.
  ▪ Diarrhea lasting more than 14 days requires therapy beyond the self-care approach and necessitates medical referral.

■ What is the underlying cause of the diarrhea?
  ▪ Has the patient traveled recently?
  ▪ Has the patient consumed any foods that have not been properly washed or handled?
  ▪ Has the patient received any vaccinations recently?
    ▫ Rotavirus vaccinations in infants may have a mild adverse effect of diarrhea.[2]
  ▪ Does the patient have any food intolerances?

TABLE 1. Assessment of dehydration and severity of acute diarrhea

	Self-Treatable		Not Self-Treatable
	Minimal or No Dehydration	**Mild-Moderate Dehydration, Diarrhea**	**Severe Dehydration, Diarrhea**
Degree of dehydration (% loss of body weight)	<3%	3%–9%	>9%
Signs of Dehydration[a]			
Mental status	Good, alert	Normal, fatigued or restless, irritable	Apathetic, lethargic, unconscious
Thirst	Drinks normally, might refuse liquids	Thirsty, eager to drink	Drinks poorly, unable to drink
Heart rate	Normal	Normal to increased	Tachycardia, bradycardia in most severe cases
Quality of pulses	Normal	Normal to decreased	Weak, thready, impalpable
Breathing	Normal	Normal, fast	Deep
Eyes	Normal	Slightly sunken[b]	Deeply sunken[b]
Tears	Present	Decreased[b]	Absent
Mouth and tongue	Moist	Dry	Parched
Skin fold	Instant recoil	Recoil in <2 seconds	Recoil in >2 seconds
Capillary refill	Normal	Prolonged	Prolonged, minimal
Extremities	Warm	Cool	Cold, mottled, cyanotic
Urine output	Normal to decreased	Decreased[b]	Minimal[b]
Number of unformed stools/day	<3	3–5	6–9
Other signs, symptoms	Afebrile, normal blood pressure, no orthostatic changes in blood pressure or pulse	May be afebrile or may develop fever >102.2°F (39.0°C), normal blood pressure, possible mild orthostatic blood pressure or pulse changes with or without mild orthostatic-related symptoms[c], sunken fontanelle[d]	Fever >102.2°F (39.0°C), low blood pressure, dizziness, severe abdominal pain

[a] If signs of dehydration are absent, rehydration therapy is not required. Maintenance therapy and replacement of stool losses should be undertaken.
[b] Signs and symptoms experienced especially by young children.
[c] Postural (orthostatic) hypotension is defined as a drop in the systolic pressure, diastolic pressure, or both of more than 15–20 mmHg on movement from a supine to an upright position and may cause lightheadedness, dizziness, or fainting. On rising, the diastolic pressure normally remains the same or increases slightly, and the systolic pressure drops slightly. If the blood pressure drops, the pulse should be checked simultaneously; the pulse rate should increase as blood pressure drops. Failure of the pulse to rise suggests the problem is neurogenic (e.g., diabetic patients with peripheral neuropathy) or that the patient may be taking a beta blocker. The presence of orthostatic hypotension suggests that the patient has lost ≥1 L of vascular volume, and referral for medical care is necessary.
[d] Signs and symptoms of concern for young infants.

● *Physical Assessment Techniques*

■ Assess skin turgor and moistness of oral mucous membranes to determine the degree of dehydration.

■ Obtain vital signs (e.g., pulse, temperature, respiratory rate, blood pressure, weight).

● ● Qu❸ST: Establish that the patient is an appropriate self-care candidate

Utilize the information collected in the patient assessment with the treatment algorithm and exclusions for self-care to determine if self-care is appropriate.

● *Exclusions to Self-Care*

Review the treatment algorithm and exclusions for self-care provided at the beginning of the chapter. This section highlights key exclusion criteria.

● *Medications*

■ See Table 2 for a list of common drug interactions.

TABLE 2. Clinically important drug-drug interactions with nonprescription antidiarrheal agents

Antidiarrheal	Drug	Potential Interaction	Management, Preventive Measures
BSS	Carbonic anhydrase inhibitors (acetazolamide, methazolamide, etc.)[a]	Increased risk for severe metabolic acidosis, salicylate toxicity, or both	Avoid high-dose salicylate therapy; if concurrent administration is necessary, monitor closely for toxicity.
BSS	Fluoroquinolones (systemic)	Decreased fluoroquinolone effectiveness	Avoid concurrent use; if concurrent use cannot be avoided, fluoroquinolone should be taken at least 2–3 hours before BSS dose. Monitor for antibiotic efficacy.
BSS	Insulin[b]	Increased risk of hypoglycemia	Monitor glucose levels more frequently and adjust insulin dose, if necessary.
BSS	Methotrexate	Increased risk of methotrexate toxicity	Avoid salicylate therapy within 10 days of high-dose methotrexate; if concurrent administration is necessary, monitor closely for toxicity.

(continued)

TABLE 2. Clinically important drug-drug interactions with nonprescription antidiarrheal agents *(Continued)*

Antidiarrheal	Drug	Potential Interaction	Management, Preventive Measures
BSS	Pramlintide	Increased risk of hypoglycemia	Monitor glucose levels more frequently and adjust insulin dose, if necessary.
BSS	Probenecid	Increased risk of hyperuricemia	Avoid persistent high-dose salicylate therapy; occasional small doses are not clinically significant.
BSS	Sulfinpyrazone	Increased risk of hyperuricemia	Avoid persistent high-dose salicylate therapy; occasional small doses are not clinically significant.
BSS	Tamarind	Increased risk of salicylate toxicity	Avoid concurrent use, if possible.
BSS	Tetracyclines (systemic)	Decreased tetracycline effectiveness	Avoid concurrent use; if concurrent use cannot be avoided, tetracycline should be taken at least 2–3 hours before BSS dose. Monitor for antibiotic efficacy.
BSS	Warfarin	Increased risk of bleeding	Avoid concurrent use, if possible. Monitor international normalized ratio closely whenever BSS is added or discontinued and adjust warfarin dose as necessary.
Loperamide	Eliglustat	Increased loperamide concentrations with enhanced central effects	Avoid concurrent use. If concurrent use cannot be avoided, monitor for loperamide adverse effects.
Loperamide	Lomitapide	Increased loperamide concentrations with enhanced central effects	Avoid concurrent use. If concurrent use cannot be avoided, monitor for loperamide adverse effects.
Loperamide	Nilotinib	Increased loperamide concentrations with enhanced central effects	Avoid concurrent use. If concurrent use cannot be avoided, monitor for loperamide adverse effects.
Loperamide	Saquinavir	Decreased saquinavir plasma concentrations	Avoid concurrent use.
Loperamide	Simeprevir	Increased loperamide concentrations with enhanced central effects	Avoid concurrent use. If concurrent use cannot be avoided, monitor for loperamide adverse effects.
Loperamide	St. John's wort	Increased risk of delirium with confusion, agitation, and disorientation	Monitor for signs of altered mental status.
Loperamide	Valerian	Increased risk of delirium with confusion, agitation, and disorientation	Monitor for signs of altered mental status.

[a]Although this interaction has not been reported with ocular carbonic anhydrase inhibitors, the possibility of an interaction should be considered.
[b]Including insulin, insulin lispro, insulin aspart, recombinant, insulin glulisine, insulin detemir, insulin degludec.

■ Conditions

- Patients who are immunocompromised, have diabetes, have severe cardio-vascular disease, or have renal disorders may have significant complications from diarrhea or dehydration, and medical referral is needed.

- Orthostatic hypotension may indicate that a patient has lost 1 L or more of vascular volume and medical referral is necessary.

- Patients, especially those over 50 years of age, with severe abdominal pain or cramping, abdominal tenderness, or distention may have a complicating acute abdominal process, such as ischemic bowel disease, and should be referred for medical evaluation.

■ Special Populations

- Self-care during pregnancy is not appropriate, as diarrhea may be due to a GI infection and potential perinatal death.

- Young infants (e.g., age of <6 months or weight of <17.5 lb) as well as those 6 months of age and older with a fever of 102.2°F or higher must be referred. Children younger than 5 years are at greater risk for complications than older children or adults because of dehydration leading to circulatory collapse and renal failure. Symptoms of dehydration in children include behavioral or mental changes (irritability, apathy, lethargy, unconscious), not having urinated in 8 hours, or having no tears when crying.

- Patients 65 years of age and older have a higher risk of death and are associated with more severe diarrhea symptoms compared to other adults.

■ ■ QuEST: Suggest appropriate self-care strategies

Select the appropriate treatment option based on the previously collected patient data. Various treatment options are discussed along with clinical pearls and pertinent patient considerations for optimal management.

■ Treatment Options

Mild-moderate dehydration from diarrhea treatment of choice is fluid and electrolyte replacement with oral rehydration solutions (ORS).

- Oral Rehydration Solutions
  - Oral treatment may be carried out in two phases: rehydration therapy and maintenance therapy.
    - Rehydration over 3–4 hours quickly replaces water and electrolyte deficits to restore normal body composition. If a child is vomiting, it is recommended to give 5 mL of ORS every few minutes.
    - Maintenance provides electrolyte solution to maintain normal body composition until adequate dietary intake is reestablished.
  - All available premixed solutions are equally safe and effective.
  - Sports drinks may be used in patients older than 5 years of age if additional sources of sodium, such as crackers or pretzels, are used concomitantly.
  - For adults who can maintain an adequate fluid intake, fluid and electrolyte status can be maintained by increasing intake of fluids, such as clear juices, soups, or sports drinks.

CAUTIONS FOR ORAL REHYDRATION SOLUTIONS

- Improper mixing of ORS dry powders by caregivers has led to fluid and electrolyte complications and injury.

Diarrhea can be treated with loperamide or bismuth subsalicylate (BSS), provided there are no contraindications.

- Loperamide
  - The American College of Gastroenterology (ACG) recommends loperamide be used for a maximum of 48 hours.
  - Adverse effects associated with loperamide include occasional dizziness and constipation. Rare adverse effects include abdominal pain, abdominal distension, nausea, vomiting, dry mouth, fatigue, and hypersensitivity reactions.

CAUTIONS FOR LOPERAMIDE

- There are reports of overdoses and cardiovascular-related deaths associated with the abuse of loperamide in individuals addicted to opioids.
- High doses of loperamide with interacting medications, such as ranitidine, cimetidine, certain macrolides (erythromycin, clarithromycin), antifungals (itraconazole, ketoconazole), and ritonavir, may increase the risk of cardiovascular events. Monitoring for loperamide adverse effects when used with a P-glycoprotein inhibitor is recommended.

- Bismuth Subsalicylate (BSS)
    - BSS is the preferred agent when vomiting is the predominant clinical symptom of acute gastroenteritis.
    - Adverse effects associated with BSS include harmless black staining of stool and darkening of the tongue.

CAUTIONS FOR BISMUTH SUBSALICYLATE

- Patients allergic to aspirin should not use BSS.
- BSS is approved for patients 12 years of age and older. Reye's syndrome is rare but can occur.
- Mild tinnitus, a dose-related adverse effect, may be associated with salicylate toxicity.
- If a patient is taking aspirin or other salicylate-containing drugs, toxic levels of salicylate may be reached even if the patient follows dosing directions on the label for each medication.
- BSS is not recommended in pregnant or nursing women or patients with bleeding risk.
- BSS should not be recommended if the patient is also taking tetracycline, quinolones, or medicines for gout (e.g., uricosurics).
- BSS should not be recommended for patients with AIDS.

Lactase deficiency prevention and treatment of diarrhea symptoms treatment of choice is lactase enzyme preparations.

- Lactase Enzyme Preparations
    - May be taken with milk or other dairy products to prevent diarrhea symptoms
    - Lactase enzyme preparations are well tolerated and are not associated with adverse effects.

Other Treatment Considerations

- Specialty diets such as the BRAT diet (e.g., bananas, rice, applesauce, toast) are not recommended, as the diet provides insufficient calories, protein, and fat, especially in situations of strict or prolonged use.

- Complementary Therapy
    - Studies have shown that probiotics, including several *Lactobacillus* species, *Bifidobacterium lactis*, and *Saccharomyces boulardii*, may be effective in preventing and treating mild, acute, uncomplicated

diarrhea. However, the Food and Drug Administration restricts claims related to these results.

- ☐ See Appendix 6 for information about common probiotics.

■ Recent studies have found zinc supplementation to be of no benefit in developed countries where zinc deficiency is rare; therefore, its use is not recommended.

● Special Populations

■ Pregnancy
  - ▪ Both loperamide and BSS are classified as Pregnancy Category C drugs. Specifically, BSS-containing products are contraindicated during the third trimester of pregnancy, as it may cause premature closure of the fetal ductus arteriosus.

■ Breastfeeding
  - ▪ Breastfeeding women should generally avoid BSS.

■ Pediatric Patients
  - ▪ For infants and children 5 years of age and younger, self-treatment is limited to treating dehydration with ORS; no antidiarrheal drugs have been shown to significantly improve clinical outcomes of acute, non-specific diarrhea in this age population.
  - ▪ Early refeeding in addition to maintenance ORS improves outcomes in children by reducing the duration of the diarrhea, reducing stool output, and improving weight gain. Current guidelines recommend withholding food no longer than 24 hours and encourage a normal, age-appropriate diet once the patient has been rehydrated, which should take no longer than 3–4 hours to accomplish. Most infants and children with acute diarrhea can tolerate full-strength breast milk and cow milk.
  - ▪ Loperamide is labeled for use in children 6 years of age and older.
  - ▪ BSS is approved for children 12 years of age and older. Reye's syndrome is rare but can occur; if children exhibit changes in behavior with nausea and vomiting, medical attention should be consulted. Children and teenagers who have or are recovering from chicken pox or flulike symptoms should not use BSS.
    - ☐ Children's Pepto antacid (calcium carbonate) is not associated with Reye's syndrome, but it is not labeled for treatment of diarrhea.

- Geriatric Patients
  - Diarrhea in older adult patients (≥65 years) is more likely to be severe and possibly fatal. Self-treatment with antidiarrheal medications should be cautioned against, and patients should be referred to a primary care provider.

◼ ◼ QuES◻: Talk with the patient

◼ *Patient Education/Counseling*

- Nonpharmacologic Talking Points
  - Continue a regular diet as tolerated; however, avoid spicy and fatty foods, foods rich in simple sugars (e.g., carbonated soft drinks, juice, gelatin desserts), and caffeine-containing beverages, which irritate the GI tract or promote fluid secretion and may worsen diarrhea.
  - Monitor weight and signs of dehydration.

- Pharmacologic Talking Points
  - Oral Rehydration Solutions
    - Counsel on appropriate volumes to administer, rates of administration, and use in vomiting.
    - Although not preferred, if using a powder ORS, provide explicit directions for mixing (use potable water) and verify understanding of the directions.
  - Loperamide
    - If abdominal distension, constipation, or ileus occurs, loperamide should be discontinued.
    - Verify age and weight to calculate an appropriate dosage and emphasize the maximum milligrams that can be taken in 24 hours:
      - Adults no more than 8 mg/day
      - Children 6–8 years no more than 4 mg/day
      - Children 9–11 years no more than 6 mg/day
  - Bismuth Subsalicylate
    - If tinnitus occurs, the product should be discontinued, and the patient should be referred for medical evaluation.
    - A darkening of the tongue may occur and may be removed by brushing the tongue with a soft-bristled brush or discontinuing the bismuth product.

- Suggest medical referral if any of the following occur:
  - If the condition remains the same or worsens after 48 hours of onset or after 72 hours of initial treatment
  - Symptoms of a high fever, bloody or mucoid stools, or signs of worsening dehydration (e.g., low blood pressure, rapid pulse, mental confusion)

Clinical Pearls

- In managing diarrhea, always look at the patient in front of you. If the patient cannot keep fluids down or looks dehydrated, they should have a medical referral.

- Many patients will seek pharmacologic treatment despite it being self-limited, but focus needs to be on rehydration.

References

1. Walker, P. Diarrhea. In: Krinsky DL, Ferreri SP, Henstreet BA, Hume AL, Newton GD, Rollins CJ, Tietze KJ, eds. *Handbook of Nonprescription Drugs: An Interactive Approach to Self-Care*. Washington, DC: American Pharmacists Association; 2017:287–308.

2. Centers for Disease Control and Prevention. Rotavirus VIS. https://www.cdc.gov/vaccines/hcp/vis/vis-statements/rotavirus.html. Accessed September 9, 2017.

EYE DISORDERS

Erin N. Adams, PharmD, BCACP

For complete information about this topic, consult Chapter 28, "Ophthalmic Disorders," written by Richard G. Fiscella and Michael K. Jensen and published in the *Handbook of Nonprescription Drugs*, 19th Edition.[1]

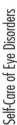

Self-Care of Eye Disorders

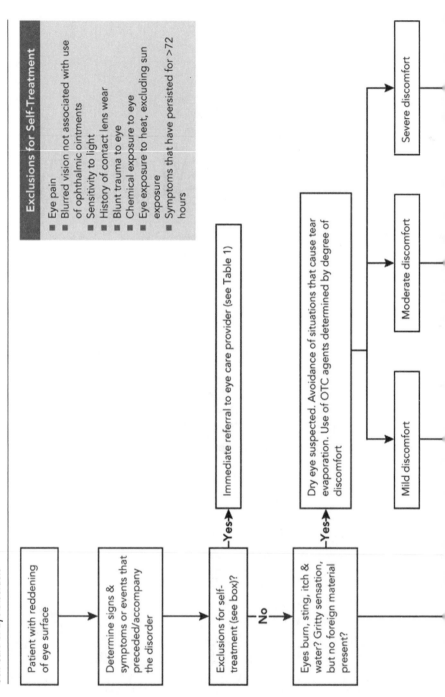

Exclusions for Self-Treatment

- Eye pain
- Blurred vision not associated with use of ophthalmic ointments
- Sensitivity to light
- History of contact lens wear
- Blunt trauma to eye
- Chemical exposure to eye
- Eye exposure to heat, excluding sun exposure
- Symptoms that have persisted for >72 hours

Patient with reddening of eye surface

↓

Determine signs & symptoms or events that preceded/accompany the disorder

↓

Exclusions for self-treatment (see box)? — **Yes→** Immediate referral to eye care provider (see Table 1)

↓ **No**

Eyes burn, sting, itch & water? Gritty sensation, but no foreign material present? — **Yes→** Dry eye suspected. Avoidance of situations that cause tear evaporation. Use of OTC agents determined by degree of discomfort

Mild discomfort   Moderate discomfort   Severe discomfort

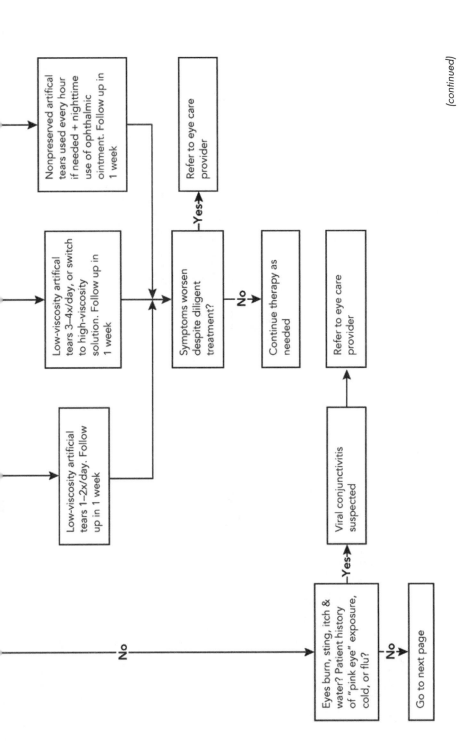

(continued)

Self-Care of Eye Disorders (*Continued*)

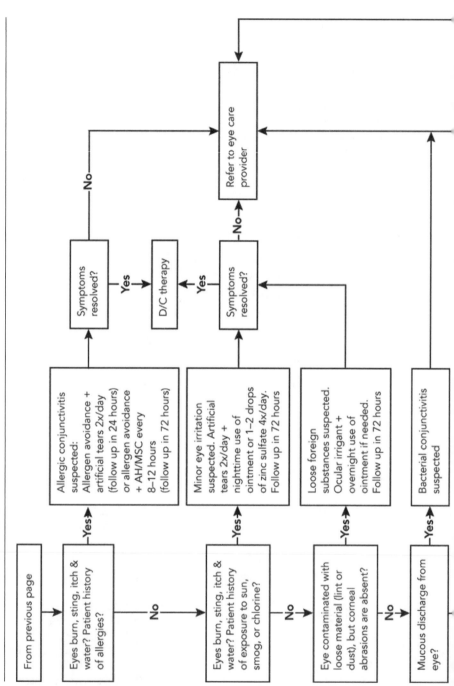

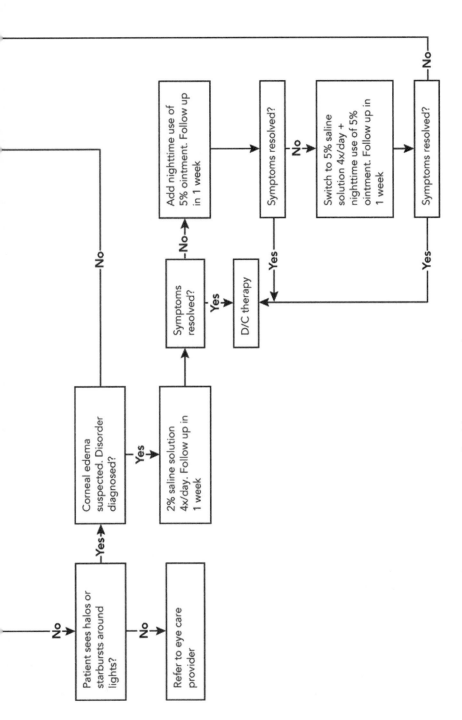

AH = antihistamine; D/C = discontinue; MSC = mast cell stabilizer; OTC = over-the-counter.

■ ■ Overview

■ Many ophthalmic disorders are self-limiting, but self-care treatment may be appropriate for some conditions that involve the eye surface, including dry eyes, allergic conjunctivitis, presence of loose foreign debris, and minor ocular irritation.

■ Goals of treatment include the following:
- For dry eyes, alleviate symptoms of irritation and prevent corneal and noncorneal tissue damage
- For allergic conjunctivitis, remove or avoid the allergen, limit or reduce the allergic reaction severity, alleviate symptoms, and protect the ocular surface
- For loose foreign substances in the eye, remove the irritant

■ ■ Pathophysiology

■ Dry eye disease is most often associated with the aging process but can also be the result of lid or corneal defects, loss of lid tissue turgor, and various conditions (e.g., thyroid disease, rheumatoid arthritis). It may be the result of suboptimal lubrication of the ocular surface and inadequate tear production. Dry eye disease is often classified into mild, moderate, and severe categories.
- Anticholinergic medications (e.g., antihistamines, antidepressants), decongestants, diuretics, and beta blockers are common agents that may cause dry eye.
- Allergens or other environmental conditions (e.g., dry or dusty working situations) or exposure to heating and air conditioning systems may contribute to dry eyes.

■ Allergic conjunctivitis is most commonly caused by pollen, animal dander, and topical eye preparations. Patients with allergic conjunctivitis also often have seasonal allergic rhinitis.

■ **Corneal edema symptoms include halos or starbursts around lights with or without changes in vision. It may occur from a variety of conditions, including overwear of contact lenses, surgical damage to the cornea, and inherited corneal dystrophies.**

▣ ▣ ⓆⓊEST: Quickly and Accurate Assess the Patient Using SCHOLAR MAC

QuEST SCHOLAR is an acronym used to assess a patient to determine self-care candidate status and to identify which treatment would be most appropriate. See Chapter 1 for a description of the QuEST SCHOLAR process.

▣ Does the Patient Have Dry or Irritated Eyes?

- Mild red eye(s) are often associated with patient complaints of discomfort, a sandy, gritty feeling, or a sensation that something is in the eye while the sclera is normal in appearance.

- Initially, dry eye disease may manifest with excessive tearing.

▣ Does the Patient Have Allergic Conjunctivitis?

- Red eye(s) with watery discharge and pruritus are common complaints.

- Vision is often not impaired but may be blurred from excessive tearing.

▣ Does the Patient Have Corneal Edema?

- Subjective perception of halos or starbursts around lights (with or without reduced vision).

- Vision is often worse upon awakening.

▣ Does the Patient Have Loose Foreign Substances in the Eye?

- The immediate symptoms are irritation, pain, tearing and feeling that something is in the eye.

▣ Does the Patient Have a Chemical Burn?

- Patients may complain of pain, irritation, photophobia, and tearing. Signs will vary according to the severity of the injury.

▣ Important SCHOLAR MAC Considerations

- Dry or irritated eyes:
    - Are the symptoms more bothersome during a certain time of day or after completing a specific activity (e.g., prolonged use of a computer screens)?

- Has the patient been outside and had overexposure to sunlight or snow blindness, which may have caused this symptom?

- Allergic conjunctivitis:
  - What exposure to allergens has the patient come into contact recently, and is there a history of seasonal allergies?

- Corneal edema:
  - Has the patient seen an ophthalmic healthcare provider already?

- Loose foreign substances in the eye:
  - Has the patient had any cuts or abrasions to the eye's surface?

Physical Assessment Techniques

- Dry or irritated eyes:
  - Inspect the patient's eyes for mild redness or irritation without sensitivity to light or trauma.

- Allergic conjunctivitis:
  - Inspect the patient for a watery discharge and red eye(s).

QuEST: Establish that the patient is an appropriate self-care candidate

Utilize the information collected in the patient assessment with the treatment algorithm and exclusions for self-care to determine if self-care is appropriate.

Exclusions to Self-Care

Review the treatment algorithm and exclusions for self-care provided at the beginning of the chapter. This section highlights key exclusion criteria.

Conditions

- Hypertension, arteriosclerosis, other cardiovascular diseases, hyperthyroidism, and diabetes could limit medication selection because of contraindications or drug-drug interactions.

- Corneal edema must be diagnosed by an ophthalmic healthcare provider before self-treatment is attempted.

■ If a foreign object or substance is embedded in the eye or trapped under the eyelid and there are abrasions on the eye's surface or the foreign substance is a fragment of wood or metal, immediate referral to an ophthalmic healthcare provider is required.

■ Chemical burns are considered a medical emergency and require immediate referral to an ophthalmic healthcare provider.

■ See Table 1 for clinical presentations of common ophthalmic conditions that require medical referral.

■ Special Populations

■ **Treatment does not vary in special populations since these are topical preparations.**

■ ■ QuE⑤T: Suggest appropriate self-care strategies

Select the appropriate treatment option based on the previously collected patient data. Various treatment options are discussed along with clinical pearls and pertinent patient considerations for optimal management.

■ Treatment Options

Eye discomfort and irritation without vision changes treatments of choice are artificial tear solutions, nonmedicated ophthalmic ointments, and mild astringents. See Table 2 for treatment recommendations for dry eye disease by severity level.

■ Artificial Tear Solutions
   ▪ Artificial tear solutions are selected based on the degree of comfort required. Increased discomfort requires a high viscosity solution (e.g., Refresh Celluvisc or Systane Ultra Preservative-Free)[2] to slow the drainage of the active ingredient from the eye, thereby increasing the retention time of the active drug and enhancing bioavailability.
   ▪ Artificial tear products without preservatives are preferred in patients with moderate-severe dry eye disease, as they are less likely to irritate the ocular surface.
   ▪ Artificial tears are not associated with adverse effects.

TABLE 1. Differentiation of ophthalmic disorders and conditions that necessitate medical referral

Disorder or Condition	Potential Signs, Symptoms	Complications	Treatment Approach
Blunt trauma	Ruptured blood vessels, bleeding into eyelid tissue space, swelling, ocular discomfort, facial drooping	Internal eye bleeding, secondary glaucoma, detached retina, periorbital bone fracture (blowout fracture)	Medical referral is appropriate.
Foreign particles trapped or embedded in the eye	Reddened eyes, profuse tearing, ocular discomfort	Corneal abrasions or scarring, chronic red eye, intraocular penetration from metal striking metal at high speeds	Medical referral for removal of particles is appropriate.
Ocular abrasions	Partial or total loss of corneal epithelium, blurred vision, profuse tearing, difficulty opening eye	Risk of bacterial or fungal infection with eye exposure to organic material, corneal scarring, anterior chamber rupture	Medical referral is appropriate.
Infections of eyelid or eye surface	Red, thickened lids, scaling, ocular discharge, matting of lashes	Scarring of lids, dry eye, corneal abrasion or scarring, loss of vision, hordeolum (stye), chalazion (risk of malignancy), blepharitis (loss of lashes, corneal irritation)	Medical referral is appropriate.
Eye exposure to chemical splash, solid chemical, or chemical fumes	Reddened eyes, watering, difficulty opening eye	Scarring of eyelids and eye surface, loss of vision	To prevent or reduce scarring of eyelids from chemical burns, flush eye immediately for at least 10 minutes, preferably with sterile saline or water. If neither is available, flush with tap water. After flushing eye, arrange immediate transportation to an emergency facility. No recommendation is noted for chemical neutralization.
Thermal injury to eye (welder's flash)	Reddened eyes, pain, sensitivity to light	Corneal scarring, secondary infection	Medical referral for definitive care (including possible eye patching) is appropriate.
Bacterial conjunctivitis	Reddened eyes with purulent, colored (mucous) discharge; ocular discomfort; eyelids stuck together on awakening	Typically self-limited, with resolution in 2 weeks	Medical referral for treatment with topical antibiotics to clear infection more quickly is appropriate; some infections require systemic antibiotic treatment.
Viral conjunctivitis	Reddened eyes with clear or white, watery discharge; ocular discomfort; hyperemic; matting of lashes	Typically self-limited, with resolution in 2 or 3 weeks	Medical provider will monitor for corneal involvement. Treatment with topical decongestants to provide comfort is appropriate; cold compresses can be applied.
Chlamydial conjunctivitis	Watery or white or yellow mucous discharge, ocular discomfort, low-grade fever, possible blurred vision	Scarring	If infection with *Chlamydia* spp. is known or suspected, or if symptoms are too vague to rule out viral or allergic conjunctivitis, medical referral is mandatory.

TABLE 2. Treatment recommendations for dry eye disease by severity level

Mild

Education, environmental modifications

Elimination of offending topical or systemic medications

Aqueous enhancement using artificial tear substitutes, gels, or ointments

Eyelid therapy (warm compresses and eyelid hygiene)

Treatment of contributing ocular factors, such as blepharitis or meibomianitis

Moderate

Same as for mild disease, plus the following:

Anti-inflammatory agents (topical cyclosporine and corticosteroids, systemic omega-3 fatty acid supplements)

Punctal plugs

Spectacle side shields and moisture chambers

Severe

Same as for mild-moderate disease, plus the following:

Systemic cholinergic agonists

Systemic anti-inflammatory agents

Mucolytic agents

Autologous serum tears

Contact lenses

Correction of eyelid abnormalities

Permanent punctal occlusion

Tarsorrhaphy

CAUTIONS FOR ARTIFICIAL TEAR SOLUTIONS

- Nonpreserved products should be discarded immediately after being opened and used, because the remaining product in the opened container can become contaminated.
- Polyvinyl alcohol can thicken or gel when used with other compounds (e.g., sodium bicarbonate, sodium borate, sulfates of sodium, potassium, zinc) and therefore is not recommended if multiple ophthalmic preparations are used, including contact lens wetting solutions.

- Nonmedicated Ophthalmic Ointments
    - The principal advantage of nonmedicated ointments is their longer retention time in the eye, which may enhance the integrity of the tear film.
    - Preservative-free, nonmedicated ointments should be recommended to avoid potential problems associated with preservatives, since they can be toxic to ocular tissues.

- Because ointments can cause blurred vision with vision limitations, combination therapy using artificial tears and nonmedicated ointments is usually recommended.
- Adverse effects include blurred vision.

> ### CAUTIONS FOR NONMEDICATED OPHTHALMIC OINTMENTS
> - Hypersensitivity reactions may occur likely from preservatives. Changing to a preservative-free formulation may eliminate these reactions.

- **Mild Astringents**
  - Zinc sulfate may be recommended for temporary relief if artificial tear solutions and nonmedicated ointments do not alleviate symptoms.
  - Astringents are typically found in combination products.

Pruritus treatment of choice is artificial tear solutions, and if symptoms persist, switch to an ophthalmic antihistamine and mast cell stabilizer. An oral antihistamine can be added, if needed.

- **Ophthalmic Antihistamine and Mast Cell Stabilizer**
  - Ketotifen provides relief within minutes, and the duration may last up to 12 hours.
  - Does not contain a vasoconstrictor, and therefore, rebound conjunctival hyperemia is not of concern
  - Adverse effects include burning, stinging, and discomfort upon instillation.

> ### CAUTIONS FOR OPHTHALMIC ANTIHISTAMINE AND MAST CELL STABILIZER
> - Contraindicated in patients with a known risk for angle-closure glaucoma
> - Ophthalmic antihistamines have anticholinergic properties and may cause pupillary dilation, which is commonly seen in patients with light-colored irises or compromised corneas (e.g., contact lens wearers) and can lead to angle-closure glaucoma.

- **Ophthalmic Antihistamine and Ocular Decongestant**
  - Although ocular antihistamines are effective alone, nonprescription products containing them also contain a decongestant and have been shown to be more effective than using either agent alone.

- Ocular decongestants should not be used for more than 72 hours, otherwise rebound conjunctival hyperemia may occur.
- Adverse effects associated with ophthalmic antihistamines include burning, stinging, and discomfort upon instillation. Ocular decongestants are generally well tolerated and do not induce ocular or systemic adverse effects.

CAUTIONS FOR OPHTHALMIC ANTIHISTAMINE AND OCULAR DECONGESTANT

- Contraindicated in patients with a known risk for angle-closure glaucoma
- Ophthalmic antihistamines have anticholinergic properties and may cause pupillary dilation, which is commonly seen in patients with light-colored irises or compromised corneas (e.g., contact lens wearers) and can lead to angle-closure glaucoma.
- Use ocular decongestants cautiously in patients with systemic hypertension, arteriosclerosis, other cardiovascular diseases, or diabetes. Adverse cardiovascular events are also possible when they are used in patients with hyperthyroidism.
- Solutions that have been stored at high temperatures may cause ocular reactions and severe mydriatic responses upon instillation.
- Ingestion of these products can result in coronary emergencies and death.

Ocular redness treatments of choice are an alpha-2 adrenergic agonist, ophthalmic decongestants, or an ophthalmic antihistamine and mast cell stabilizer.

- **Alpha-2 Adrenergic Agonist**
    - Brimonidine is the first and only nonprescription ophthalmic drop that contains a low-dose alpha-2 adrenergic agoinst.[3]
    - Onset is approximately 1 minute with duration of action up to 8 hours.[3]
    - Adverse effects associated with ophthalmic brimonidine include burning, itching of the eye, and conjunctival discoloration.[4]

CAUTIONS FOR ALPHA-2 ADRENERGIC AGONISTS

- Do not use if eye pain, changes in vision, continued redness, or irritation of the eye occur.

■ Ophthalmic Decongestants
  ▪ Will decrease ocular redness but will not diminish the allergic response
  ▪ Ocular decongestants should not be used for more than 72 hours, otherwise rebound conjunctival hyperemia may occur.
  ▪ Rebound congestion appears to be less likely with topical ocular use of naphazoline or tetrahydrozoline.
  ▪ Ocular decongestants are generally well tolerated and do not induce ocular or systemic adverse effects.

CAUTIONS FOR OPHTHALMIC DECONGESTANTS

- Contraindicated in patients with a known risk for angle-closure glaucoma
- Use ocular decongestants cautiously in patients with systemic hypertension, arteriosclerosis, other cardiovascular diseases, or diabetes. Adverse cardiovascular events are also possible when they are used in patients with hyperthyroidism.
- Ingestion of these products can result in coronary emergencies and death.

Eye discomfort with vision changes treatment of choice is topical hyperosmotics after diagnosis of corneal edema from an ophthalmic healthcare provider.

■ Hyperosmotics
  ▪ Only sodium chloride can be obtained without a prescription in both solution and ointment formulations.
  ▪ Several drops during the first few waking hours may be beneficial, since symptoms are often worse upon awakening.
  ▪ Initial treatment is instillation of the 2% solution, and if symptoms persist for more than 1–2 weeks, nighttime use of the 5% ointment should be added to the regimen. If symptoms persist after titration, the patient should switch to a higher percentage solution and continue nighttime use of the ointment.
  ▪ Adverse effects associated with hyperosmotics include stinging and burning, especially with higher strength ointments. The ointment is reserved for nighttime administration to avoid blurred vision.

CAUTIONS FOR HYPEROSMOTICS

- Contraindicated in patients with a traumatic injury of the corneal epithelium
- To avoid adverse effects with chronic use, patients should use a lower strength of hyperosmotics.
- Caution patients against preparation of homemade saline solutions for use in the eye because of the associated risk of infection.

Eye discomfort with vision changes treatments of choice are ocular irrigants and, if needed, a nonmedicated ophthalmic ointment to provide prolonged duration of protection.

- Ocular Irrigants
  - Used to cleanse ocular tissues or to clear away unwanted ocular debris while maintaining moisture
  - Ocular irrigants are not associated with adverse effects.

CAUTIONS FOR OCULAR IRRIGANTS

- Do not use for open wounds in or near the eyes.

- Complementary Therapy
  - Similasan Dry Eye Relief eye drops, which contain *Atropa belladonnabelladonna*, *Euphrasia*, and *Mercurius sublimatus*, are marketed to relieve dryness and redness caused by smog, contact lens wear, and other factors. The efficacy of this formulation has not been established in controlled clinical trials.
  - Omega-3 oils or flaxseed oil supplementation with the recommended doses by the manufacturer are thought to improve lid function with dry eye, possibly from anti-inflammatory properties.
  - Similasan Allergy Eye Relief eye drops, which contain *Apis*, *Euphrasia*, and sabadilla, are indicated for relief from itching and burning caused by allergic reactions. The efficacy of this formulation has not been established in controlled clinical trials.

■ Special Populations

■ Pregnancy

▪ During pregnancy, women should use ocular decongestants sparingly, if at all.

■ Pediatric Patients

▪ Ketotifen, an ophthalmic antihistamine and mast cell stabilizer, is approved for patients 3 years of age and older; otherwise, the approach to treating is the same as that for the general population.

■ Geriatric Patients

▪ Older adult patients with a known risk for angle-closure glaucoma are not appropriate candidates for self-care with ocular antihistamines.

▪ Older adult patients with hypertension, arteriosclerosis, other cardio-vascular diseases, diabetes, or hyperthyroidism are cautioned from using ocular decongestants.

■ ■ QuES❶: Talk with the patient

■ Patient Education/Counseling

■ Nonpharmacologic Talking Points

▪ Eye Discomfort and Irritation without Vision Changes

▫ Discontinue any offending agents and avoid environments or activities that are known to cause eye discomfort and irritation.

▫ Application of warm compresses and use of a humidifier may increase eye comfort.

▫ Recommend repositioning workstations away from heating and air conditioning vents.

▫ Wearing eye protection (e.g., sunglasses, goggles) in windy, out-door environments may further help alleviate and prevent symptoms in the future. Maintain good eyelid hygiene.

▪ Ocular Redness

▫ Removal or avoidance of the responsible allergen is the best treatment. It is recommended to check the pollen count, keep doors and windows closed, run air conditioning, and use air filters to help decrease allergen triggers.

▫ Applying cold compresses 3–4 times a day may help reduce redness and itching.

▫ Contact lenses should not be used until the allergic symptoms resolve.

- Eye Discomfort with Vision Changes
  - Avoid rubbing the affected eye. If reflex tearing does not remove the foreign material, flush the eyes with copious amounts of water from a faucet or garden hose.

- Pharmacologic Talking Points
  - Ophthalmic Administration
    - Proper drug instillation technique is critical if the eye is to receive the maximum benefit from the medication.
    - Remove contact lenses before use and wait 10 minutes before reinserting contact lenses.
    - Wait 5 minutes before instilling other ophthalmic products.
    - See "Appendix 1: Administration Guidelines for Nasal, Ophthalmic, and Otic Dosage Formulations."
  - Discard or replace eye drop bottles 30 days after the sterility safety seal is punctured. The manufacturer's expiration date does not apply once the seal is broken.
  - Single dose products do not contain a preservative and should be discarded immediately after being opened and used.
  - Artificial Tear Solutions
    - Instilling drops at least twice daily is an appropriate initial regimen.
  - Nonmedicated Ophthalmic Ointments
    - Ointments may cause blurred vision.
    - Many patients prefer to instill the ointment at bedtime to keep the eyes moist during sleep and to help prevent morning symptoms.
  - Ophthalmic Decongestants
    - Should not be used for more than 72 hours, as rebound conjunctival hyperemia and conjunctivitis eyelid swelling may occur with prolonged use
  - Hyperosmotics
    - Counsel patients against preparation of homemade solutions for use in the eye because of the associated risk of infection.
  - Ocular Irrigants
    - To reduce the risk of contamination, patients should use ocular irrigants only on a short-term basis. Irrigants may be packaged with an eyecup; however, because contamination of the eyecup is possible, it should never be used to rinse the eye.

- Suggest medical referral if any of the following occur:
  - Symptoms persist after 72 hours in any self-treated condition
  - Patient has apparent rebound conjunctival hyperemia

- For patients with corneal edema, if titrated solutions and ointment combination therapy do not provide relief after 3 weeks, a second referral is needed.
- If a foreign object or substance becomes embedded in the eye or trapped under the eyelid, see an ophthalmic healthcare provider for removal. Medical referral is also warranted if the patient experiences unremitting eye pain, changes in vision, continued redness or irritation of the eye, or the ocular condition persists or worsens.
- Chemical burns require immediate referral to an ophthalmic healthcare provider to prevent development of conjunctival adhesions and corneal complications.

Clinical Pearls

- Nonprescription ophthalmic products should be used only in cases of minor pain or discomfort. If the nature of the problem is in doubt, the patient should be referred to an ophthalmic healthcare provider.

- Select single-entity products as much as possible to avoid complications and adverse effects, as often one agent will alleviate symptoms.

- The lowest concentration and conservative dosage frequencies should be used, especially for ocular decongestants; overuse should be avoided.

References

1. Fiscella RG, Jensen MK. Opthalmic disorders. In: Krinsky DL, Ferreri SP, Henstreet BA, Hume AL, Newton GD, Rollins CJ, Tietze KJ, eds. *Handbook of Nonprescription Drugs: An Interactive Approach to Self-Care*. Washington, DC: American Pharmacists Association; 2017:545–566.

2. Stephenson, M. OTC drops: Telling the tears apart. https://www.reviewofophthalmology.com/article/otc-drops-telling-the-tears-apart. Accessed June 13, 2018.

3. Bausch+Lomb. Lumify Redness Reliever Eye Drops. http://www.bausch.com/ecp/our-products/otc-ophthalmics/lumify-drops. Accessed June 5, 2018.

4. Anon. Brimonidine tartrate, adverse effects. DRUGDEX® System (electronic version). http://www.micromedexsolutions.com. Accessed June 17, 2018.

5. Scolaro, KL. Colds and allergy. In: Krinsky DL, Ferreri SP, Henstreet BA, Hume AL, Newton GD, Rollins CJ, Tietze KJ, eds. *Handbook of Nonprescription Drugs: An Interactive Approach to Self-Care*. Washington, DC: American Pharmacists Association; 2017:189–216.

FEVER

Connie Kang, PharmD, BCPS, BCGP

For complete information about this topic, consult Chapter 6, "Fever," written by Virginia Lemay and Brett Feret and published in the *Handbook of Nonprescription Drugs*, 19th Edition.[1]

Self-Care of Fever

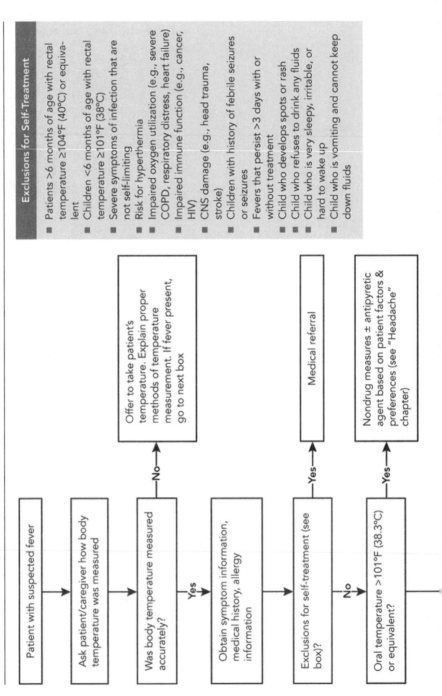

Exclusions for Self-Treatment

- Patients >6 months of age with rectal temperature ≥104°F (40°C) or equivalent
- Children <6 months of age with rectal temperature ≥101°F (38°C)
- Severe symptoms of infection that are not self-limiting
- Risk for hyperthermia
- Impaired oxygen utilization (e.g., severe COPD, respiratory distress, heart failure)
- Impaired immune function (e.g., cancer, HIV)
- CNS damage (e.g., head trauma, stroke)
- Children with history of febrile seizures or seizures
- Fevers that persist >3 days with or without treatment
- Child who develops spots or rash
- Child who refuses to drink any fluids
- Child who is very sleepy, irritable, or hard to wake up
- Child who is vomiting and cannot keep down fluids

Patient with suspected fever

Ask patient/caregiver how body temperature was measured

Was body temperature measured accurately? — **No** → Offer to take patient's temperature. Explain proper methods of temperature measurement. If fever present, go to next box

↓ **Yes**

Obtain symptom information, medical history, allergy information

Exclusions for self-treatment (see box)? — **Yes** → Medical referral

↓ **No**

Oral temperature >101°F (38.3°C) or equivalent? — **Yes** → Nondrug measures ± antipyretic agent based on patient factors & preferences (see "Headache" chapter)

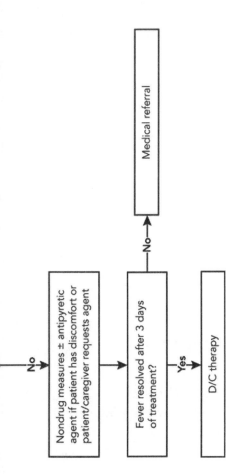

CNS = central nervous system; COPD = chronic obstructive pulmonary disease; D/C = discontinue; HIV = human immunodeficiency virus.

■ ■ Overview

■ Fever is symptomatic of a larger underlying process (e.g., infection, abnormal metabolism, drug-induced) that should be identified and treated appropriately.

■ Fever may be of physiologic benefit. Most fevers are self-limiting and non-threatening; however, fever can cause a great deal of discomfort (e.g., generalized malaise, myalgia, arthralgia, headache, tachycardia, diaphoresis, chills, irritability, anorexia).

■ Fevers rarely poses serious health concerns, unless greater than 106.4°F (41.1°C).

■ The goal of self-treatment with antipyretic therapy is not to normalize temperature but to improve overall comfort and well-being.

■ ■ Pathophysiology

■ Normal thermoregulation prevents wide fluctuations in body temperature; the average oral temperature is 97.5°F-98.9°F (36.4°C–37.2°C). This is the "set point" at which physiologic or behavioral mechanisms are not activated. The commonly accepted core body temperature is usually an oral measurement of 98.6°F (37.0°C).

■ Core body temperature is controlled by the hypothalamus and regulated by a feedback system. Skin temperature can fluctuate greatly in response to environmental conditions, while the core temperature is regulated within a narrow range.

■ Fever is caused by a regulated rise in body temperature in response to a pyrogen. Pyrogens activate the body's host defenses, resulting in an increase in the set point, which increases the core temperature.

■ Prostaglandins are produced in response to circulating pyrogens and elevate the thermoregulatory set point. Within hours, body temperature reaches the new set point and fever occurs. The patient will likely experience chills caused by peripheral vasoconstriction and muscle rigidity to maintain homeostasis.

■ ■ ⓆⓊEST: Quickly and Accurate Assess the Patient Using SCHOLAR MAC

QuEST SCHOLAR is an acronym used to assess a patient to determine self-care candidate status and to identify which treatment would be most appropriate. See Chapter 1 for a description of the QuEST SCHOLAR process.

■ Does the Patient Have a Fever?

- The most important sign of a fever is an elevated temperature.

- Table 1 provides temperatures at which a patient can be assessed as having a fever based on location.

- Fevers are symptomatic presentations of a larger underlying process, such as an infection or drug-induced fever. Potential causes should be investigated.

- Signs and symptoms that typically accompany fever include headache, diaphoresis, generalized malaise, chills, tachycardia, arthralgia, myalgia, irritability, and anorexia.

- Children can tolerate fever well, and fever is generally of minor concern if the child is alert, playing normally, and staying hydrated.

- High body temperature dulls intellectual function and can cause delirium and disorientation.

■ Important SCHOLAR MAC Considerations

- Is the measured temperature accurate?
  - Oral temperature measurement should be taken at least 30 minutes after eating or drinking.

TABLE 1. Body temperature range based on site of measurement

Site of Measurement	Normal Range[a]	Fever[a]
Rectal	97.9°F–100.4°F (36.6°C–38.0°C)	>100.4°F (38.0°C)
Oral	95.9°F–99.5°F (35.5°C–37.5°C)	>99.5°F (37.5°C)
Axillary	94.5°F–99.3°F (34.7°C–37.4°C)	>99.3°F (37.4°C)
Tympanic	96.3°F–100.0°F (35.7°C–37.8°C)	>100.0°F (37.8°C)
Temporal	97.9°F–100.1°F (36.6°C–37.8°C)	0–2 months of age: >100.7°F (38.1°C) 3–47 months of age: >100.3°F (37.9°C) >4 years of age: >100.1°F (37.8°C)

[a]Conversion formulas: Celsius = 5/9(°F − 32); Fahrenheit = (9/5 × °C) + 32.

- If fever was detected via the less reliable axillary method, confirmation using another method is recommended.
- Consider asking the patient or caregiver to describe which thermometer was used and how it was used. Correct technique is described in Appendix 2.

■ Has an antipyretic been taken? How long after administration was the temperature measured?
  - It is important to know whether a fever is treated or not. Fever cutoffs for medical referral vs. self-treatment reflect untreated temperatures.
  - Antipyretics will typically lower temperature by 1°F-2°F.
  - This reduction should be factored into decisions about whether self-treatment is appropriate or medical referral is needed when a reported temperature is treated.

■ What symptoms of fever (i.e., discomfort) are the patient experiencing and how severe are they?
  - This can help guide product selection, dosing, and supportive care.

● Physical Assessment Techniques

■ Feeling a part of the body may identify an increase in skin temperature but does not accurately detect a rise in core temperature.

■ A thermometer must be used to measure the core temperature for accurate fever detection. Core temperature can be estimated using various types of thermometers at the rectal, oral, axillary, tympanic, or temporal sites.

■ Body temperature should be measured with the same thermometer at the same site throughout the course of an illness, since readings from different thermometers or body sites may vary. Table 1 details normal and fever body temperature ranges based on the site of measurement.
  - Individual body temperature may differ by 1.8°F-2.5°F (1.0°C-1.4°C) from these norms.
  - Diurnal rhythms cause body temperature to vary during the day, with higher temperatures typically occurring in the late afternoon to early evening.

■ Estimate temperature equivalency between sites using the following simplified conversion:
  - Add 1°F to an oral temperature for a rectal, tympanic, or temporal equivalent.
  - Subtract 1°F from an oral temperature for an axillary equivalent.

- Some thermometers can be set to automatically convert and display the measured temperature as a rectal or oral temperature equivalent.

- Appendix 2 provides a thorough review of available thermometer products.
  - Rectal temperature is the preferred measurement site up to 3 months of age.
  - Tympanic temperature should not be used in patients younger than 6 months of age.

▆ ▆ QuⒺST: Establish that the patient is an appropriate self-care candidate

Utilize the information collected in the patient assessment with the treatment algorithm and exclusions for self-care to determine if self-care is appropriate.

▆ Exclusions to Self-Care

Review the treatment algorithm and exclusions for self-care provided at the beginning of the chapter. This section highlights key factors.

▆ Medications

- Table 2 provides important drug-drug interactions to consider for nonprescription analgesics and antipyretics.
  - Warfarin—potential treatment options can increase risk of bleeding. Acetaminophen likely does not affect international normalized ratio (INR) if less than 2 g/day.
  - Alcohol—patients consuming 3 or more drinks/day are at greatest risk for hepatotoxicity.

- Fevers can be caused by medication use, and the febrile response to the administration of a medication is referred to as drug fever. Medications known to cause drug fever include amphetamines, antibiotics, antineoplastics, antipsychotics, illicit drugs, tricyclic antidepressants (TCAs).

▆ Conditions

- Dementia, cerebrovascular arteriosclerosis, and alcoholism—risk of delirium and disorientation with high body temperature. Antipyretic use for fever should be carefully considered based on renal and hepatic function. May consider medical referral sooner.

TABLE 2. Clinically important drug-drug interactions with nonprescription analgesic agents

Analgesic, Antipyretic	Drug	Potential Interaction	Management and Preventive Measures
Acetaminophen	Alcohol	Increased risk of hepatotoxicity	Avoid concurrent use if possible; minimize alcohol intake when using acetaminophen.
Acetaminophen	Warfarin	Increased risk of bleeding (elevations in INR)	Limit acetaminophen to occasional use; monitor INR for several weeks when acetaminophen 2–4 g daily is added or discontinued in patients on warfarin.
Aspirin	Valproic acid	Displacement from protein-binding sites and inhibition of valproic acid metabolism	Avoid concurrent use; use naproxen instead of aspirin (no interaction).
Aspirin	NSAIDs, including COX-2 inhibitors	Increased risk of gastroduodenal ulcers and bleeding	Avoid concurrent use if possible.
Ibuprofen	Aspirin	Decreased antiplatelet effect of aspirin	Aspirin should be taken at least 30 minutes before or 8 hours after ibuprofen. Use acetaminophen (or other analgesic) instead of ibuprofen.
Ibuprofen	Phenytoin	Displacement from protein-binding sites	Monitor free phenytoin levels; adjust dose as indicated.
NSAIDs	Bisphosphonates	Increased risk of GI or esophageal ulceration	Use caution with concomitant use.
NSAIDs	Digoxin	Renal clearance of digoxin inhibited	Monitor digoxin levels; adjust dose as indicated.
Salicylates and NSAIDs	Antihypertensive agents, beta blockers, ACE inhibitors, vaso-dilators, diuretics	Antihypertensive effect inhibited; possible hyperkalemia with potassium-sparing diuretics and ACE inhibitors	Monitor blood pressure, cardiac function, and potassium levels.
Salicylates and NSAIDs	Anticoagulants	Increased risk of bleeding, especially GI	Avoid concurrent use if possible; risk is lowest with salsalate and choline magnesium trisalicylate.
Salicylates and NSAIDs	Alcohol	Increased risk of GI bleeding	Avoid concurrent use, if possible; minimize alcohol intake when using salicylates and NSAIDs.
Salicylates and NSAIDs	Methotrexate	Decreased methotrexate clearance	Avoid salicylates and NSAIDs with high-dose methotrexate therapy; monitor levels with concurrent treatment.
Salicylates (moderate-high doses)	Sulfonylureas	Increased risk of hypoglycemia	Avoid concurrent use if possible; monitor blood glucose levels when changing salicylate dose.

Abbreviations used: ACE, angiotensin-converting enzyme; COX, cyclooxygenase.

- Cardiovascular diseases (e.g., heart failure, high blood pressure, previous heart attack) can be worsened by nonsteroidal anti-inflammatory drug (NSAID) use. Short-term use for fever symptoms is likely okay.

- NSAIDs should be used cautiously in patients with renal dysfunction.

- Acetaminophen should be used cautiously in patients with hepatic dysfunction.

Special Populations

- Infants under 3 months of age whose rectal temperatures are 100.4°F (38.0°C) or greater should be referred to their pediatrician or an urgent care or emergency room. Their immature immune systems are prone to more serious bacterial infections.
  - Provide self-care measures while medical evaluation is being sought.

- Febrile seizures should be referred to a pediatrician for evaluation.

- Any child with a rectal temperature of 104.0°F (40.0°C) or greater should be referred to a pediatrician.

- Aspirin-containing products should not be used in children under 16 years of age with viral illnesses because of the risk of Reye's syndrome.

- Older adults (≥65 years of age) should cautiously use NSAIDs, as they are included in the 2015 Updated Beers Criteria. Short-term use is likely less problematic.

- Older adults are at a higher risk for fever-related complications because of decreased thirst perception and ability to perspire. These patients should be carefully monitored for worsening condition.

QuEST: Suggest appropriate self-care strategies

Select the appropriate treatment option based on the previously collected patient data. Various treatment options are discussed along with clinical pearls and pertinent patient considerations for optimal management.

Treatment Options

Fever treatment of choice is a single-entity antipyretic.

- Acetaminophen
  - It is unclear whether acetaminophen or NSAIDs (e.g., ibuprofen) are superior in treating fever based on inconsistent clinical trial findings.

Data suggest ibuprofen may provide a slight benefit with a quicker onset and longer duration of action.

- Adverse effects associated with acetaminophen include nausea, hepatotoxicity, and skin rash (rare). It is well-tolerated when recommended doses are not exceeded.

CAUTIONS FOR ACETAMINOPHEN

- Acetaminophen is potentially hepatotoxic in doses exceeding 4 g/day, especially with chronic use.
- The FDA recommends an acetaminophen maximum daily dosage of 3000–3250 mg to lower the risk of accidental acetaminophen overdose.
- More conservative dosing (≤2 g/day) or avoidance may be considered in the following patients at increased risk for acetaminophen-induced hepatotoxicity: liver disease, 3 or more alcoholic drinks/day, concurrent hepatotoxic drug(s), and poor nutritional intake.

- NSAIDs
  - Individual patients may report a better response to one NSAID than to another for reasons that are unclear. Using an alternative NSAID may be effective when patients have previously failed to get relief from an NSAID.
  - Adverse effects associated with NSAIDs include heartburn, dyspepsia, anorexia, epigastric pain, bleeding and bruising, and increased blood pressure.

CAUTIONS FOR NSAIDS

- Calculate the appropriate dose of pediatric liquid ibuprofen at each treatment course to prevent dosing errors that are possible because of the availability of two concentrations (50 mg/1.25 mL concentrated drops and 100 mg/5 mL suspension).
- NSAIDs are associated with increased serious gastrointestinal (GI; e.g., ulceration, bleeding), cardiovascular (e.g., myocardial infarction, stroke, heart failure), and nephropathy risks.
- Naproxen is considered the safer NSAID option for cardiovascular risk. Patients should take the minimum dose for the shortest duration to control symptoms.

- Salicylates
  - Aspirin may be considered for use as an antipyretic, but generally, risks outweigh benefits at the dose required for pyresis.

- Adverse effects associated with salicylates include nausea, vomiting, bleeding, and dyspepsia.

> **CAUTIONS FOR SALICYLATES**
> - Avoid aspirin in patients with risk factors for upper GI bleeding. Risk factors include age over 60 years, regular alcohol use, history of peptic ulcer, and concomitant use of NSAIDs, anticoagulants, antiplatelet agents, bisphosphonates, selective serotonin reuptake inhibitors, or systemic corticosteroids.
> - Avoid use of aspirin-containing products with uncontrolled high blood pressure, heart failure, bleeding disorders, or renal failure.
> - Avoid effervescent aspirin solutions with high sodium content in patients who have hypertension, heart failure, or renal failure.

Other Treatment Considerations

- Fever is an indicator of an underlying process. Treatment should focus on the primary cause rather than on the temperature reading.

- Complementary Therapy
    - Currently, insufficient evidence exists to recommend any dietary supplement or other complementary therapy for the treatment of fever.

Special Populations

- Pregnancy
    - Generally, NSAIDs should not be used in pregnancy unless it is clear that the potential benefit justifies the potential risk to the fetus. NSAIDs are not known to be teratogenic but can cause prolonged labor and increased postpartum bleeding. They can also cause adverse fetal cardiovascular effects (e.g., premature closing of the ductus arteriosus). Risks of use are greatest in the third trimester.
    - Acetaminophen crosses the placenta but is considered safe for pregnancy and is the first-line treatment for conditions that required oral systemic analgesics. It has long been considered safe in pregnancy, but emerging evidence suggests there may be a slight association between maternal prenatal use of acetaminophen and attention deficit hyperactivity disorder (ADHD) in the child. Duration of use that is less than 8 days is negatively associated with ADHD. Duration of use that is more than 29 days has the greatest association. Patients should be advised of this potential association; however, short-term use appears nonsignificant.[3]

- Aspirin can cross the placenta and poses both fetal and maternal harms. Thus, it should be avoided in pregnancy, particularly during the last semester.

- Breastfeeding
  - Acetaminophen appears in breast milk but is considered compatible with breastfeeding. A rarely occurring maculopapular rash in infants, which subsides with discontinuation, is the only adverse effect reported in infants exposed through breast milk.
  - Naproxen should be avoided in nursing mothers. It is unknown if ibuprofen is excreted into breastmilk. Thus, ibuprofen use should be carefully weighed against potential harm to the infant.
  - Avoid aspirin during breastfeeding because of the potential risk of affecting platelet function in nursing infants.

- Pediatric Patients
  - Children 12 years of age or younger should be dosed by body weight (mg/kg) using the table provided on the product.
    - Conversion from pounds (lb) to kilograms (kg): 2.2 lb = 1 kg.
    - Ibuprofen dose: 5–10 mg/kg every 6–8 hours.
      - Maximum of 40 mg/kg/day.
    - Acetaminophen dose: 10–15 mg/kg every 4–6 hours.
      - Maximum of 5 doses/day.
  - Naproxen is not indicated for children 12 years of age or younger.

- Geriatric Patients
  - Acetaminophen is generally recognized as the agent of choice for mild-moderate pain in older adults because of the increased risk of serious GI, cardiovascular, and renal effects of NSAIDs and salicylates.

⬛ ⬤ QuES⬤: Talk with the patient

⬤ Patient Education/Counseling

- Nonpharmacologic Talking Points
  - Monitor body temperature: use the same thermometer at the same body site 2–3 times per day.
    - Avoid excessive temperature monitoring (e.g., every hour).
  - Monitor the level of discomfort: for all levels of fever, wear light-weight clothing, remove blankets, maintain room temperature at

approximately 68.0°F (20.0°C), and drink sufficient fluid to replenish insensible losses and prevent dehydration.

◦ Increase fluid intake by at least 1–2 oz per hour in children and by at least 3–4 oz per hour in adults, unless fluids are contraindicated.

◦ Balanced electrolyte replenishment drinks (e.g., Pedialyte), water, or ice pops may be offered.

■ Exercise caution in recommending high sugar drinks (e.g., sports drinks, fruit juice) to patients with diarrhea, as the diarrhea may worsen.

■ Pharmacologic Talking Points

  ▪ Patients should be reminded of the maximum dosages of nonprescription analgesic and antipyretic treatment:

    ◦ Ibuprofen maximum dose is 1200 mg/day.

    ◦ Naproxen sodium maximum dose is 660 mg/day.

    ◦ Acetaminophen maximum dose is 3000–3250 mg/day.

  ▪ Nonprescription analgesics and antipyretics typically take ½ to 1 hour to begin to decrease discomfort and lower body temperature.

    ◦ Acetaminophen and ibuprofen show reduction of approximately 1°F-2°F within 30 minutes to 1 hour, with maximum reduction usually within 2 hours.

    ◦ Although most patients demonstrate a reduction in temperature after each individual dose of an antipyretic, nonpharmacologic therapy for fever may take a full day to result in a decrease in temperature.

  ▪ The American Academy of Pediatrics does not recommend alternating antipyretics because of the risk of overdose, medication errors resulting from the complexity of the regimens, and an increased rate of adverse effects.

    ◦ If the patient or caregiver has been instructed by a primary care provider to alternate antipyretics, encourage caregivers to log the generic name, dose, and time of administration for each medication to minimize the likelihood of duplicate dosing and adverse effects.

  ▪ To avoid incorrect dosing of liquid dosage forms, instruct caregivers to use only the calibrated measuring device provided with the medication, which should be used only with the accompanying medication.

  ▪ Completely chew chewable tablets, then drink a full glass of water.

  ▪ NSAIDs can be taken with food or milk to decrease stomach irritation.

■ Suggest medical referral if any of the following occur:

  ▪ Fever persists more than 3 days, with or without treatment, in patients 2 years of age and older

- Fever persists more than 24 hours in patients 2 years of age and younger
- Infants less than 3 months of age who experience rectal fever greater than 100.4°F (38.0°C)—but provide self-care recommendation while medical treatment is being sought
- Any patient with a fever greater than 104.0°F (40.0°C)
- If drug fever is suspected (e.g., temporal relationship between the fever and the administration of a medication)—failure to discontinue the offending drug may result in substantial morbidity and death

Clinical Pearls

- Overtreatment of fever for viral and bacterial infections may be detrimental. Fever may have beneficial effects on host defense mechanisms and impair the growth of certain pyrogens.

- Consider the patient in selecting the antipyretic and dosage form:
  - Consideration of palatability may improve outcomes and adherence in children.
  - Consideration of a more convenient dosing frequency may improve adherence, especially in children who have difficulty taking medicine.
    - Ibuprofen is administered every 6–8 hours.
    - Naproxen is administered every 12 hours.
    - Acetaminophen is administered every 4–6 hours.

References

1. Lemay V, Feret B. Fever. In: Krinsky DL, Ferreri SP, Hemstreet BA, Hume AL, Newton GD, Rollins CJ, Tietze KJ, eds. *Handbook of Nonprescription Drugs: An Interactive Approach to Self-Care*. Washington, DC: American Pharmacists Association; 2017:97–110.

2. Wilkinson JJ, Tromp K. Headache. In: Krinsky DL, Ferreri SP, Hemstreet BA, Hume AL, Newton GD, Rollins CJ, Tietze KJ, eds. *Handbook of Nonprescription Drugs: An Interactive Approach to Self-Care*. Washington, DC: American Pharmacists Association; 2017:77–96.

3. Ystrom E, Gustavson K, Brandlistuen RE, et al. Prenatal exposure to acetaminophen and risk of ADHD. *Pediatrics*. 2017;140(5):e20163840.

FUNGAL SKIN INFECTIONS

Albert Bach, PharmD

For complete information about this topic, consult Chapter 42, "Fungal Skin Infections," written by April Gardner and Natalie Walkup and published in the *Handbook of Nonprescription Drugs*, 19th Edition.[1]

Self-Care of Fungal Skin Infections

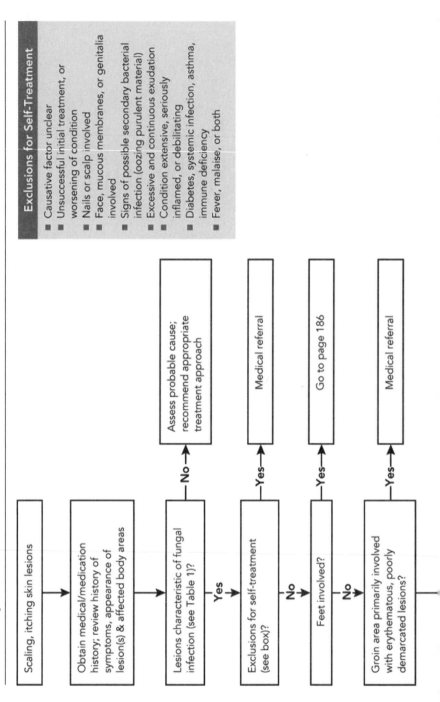

Scaling, itching skin lesions

Obtain medical/medication history; review history of symptoms, appearance of lesion(s) & affected body areas

Lesions characteristic of fungal infection (see Table 1)?

No → Assess probable cause; recommend appropriate treatment approach

Yes

Exclusions for self-treatment (see box)?

Yes → Medical referral

No

Feet involved?

Yes → Go to page 186

No

Groin area primarily involved with erythematous, poorly demarcated lesions?

Yes → Medical referral

Exclusions for Self-Treatment

- Causative factor unclear
- Unsuccessful initial treatment, or worsening of condition
- Nails or scalp involved
- Face, mucous membranes, or genitalia involved
- Signs of possible secondary bacterial infection (oozing purulent material)
- Excessive and continuous exudation
- Condition extensive, seriously inflamed, or debilitating
- Diabetes, systemic infection, asthma, immune deficiency
- Fever, malaise, or both

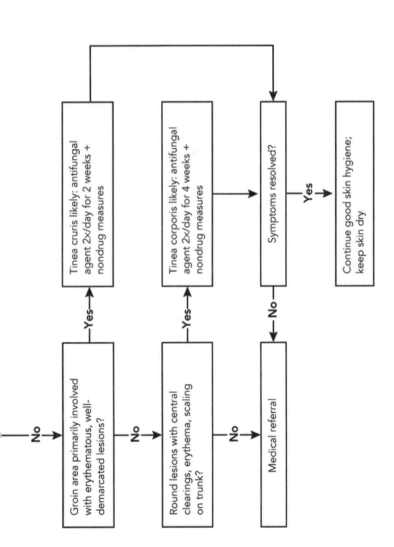

(continued)

Self-Care of Fungal Skin Infections *(Continued)*

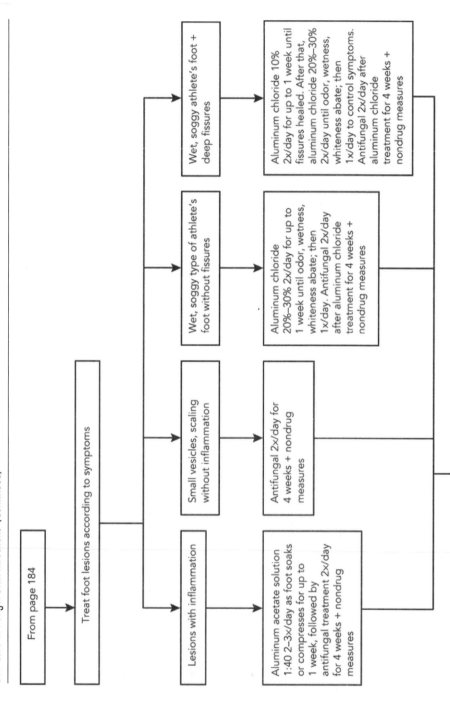

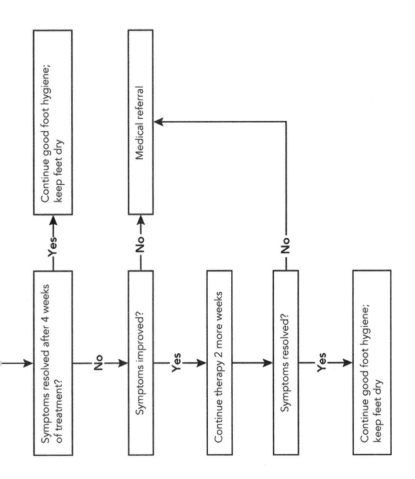

▩▩ Overview

- Infections caused by dermatophyte fungi, often referred to as tinea or ringworm, are common superficial infections that can affect the hair, skin, and nails.

- Tinea infections are named according to the area of body that is affected (e.g., scalp [tinea capitis]; groin [tinea cruris]; body [tinea corporis]; feet [tinea pedis]; nails [tinea unguium]). All but scalp and nail infections can be self-treated with nonprescription antifungals.

- The goals of treating fungal skin infections are to (1) provide symptomatic relief, (2) eradicate existing infection, and (3) prevent future infections.

▩▩ Pathophysiology

- Dermatophytes are fungi that require keratin for survival, and therefore, their infections are limited to the superficial skin, hair, and nails.

- After inoculation, the dermatophyte undergoes an incubation and enlargement stage where it grows in the superficial layer of the skin, followed by a refractory and involution stage.

- After the infection is established, the size and duration of the lesions depend on the growth rate of the organism and the epidermal turnover rate. The fungal growth rate must equal or exceed the epidermal turnover rate, or the organism will be quickly shed.

▩ *Transmission*

- Tinea infections are highly contagious and can occur through contact with infected people, animals, soil, or infected fomites (e.g., hats, combs, clothing, upholstery).

▩ *Preventative Measures*

- Keep the skin clean and dry, avoid sharing personal articles, and avoid contact with infected fomites or persons who have a fungal infection.

- Wear protective footwear (e.g., rubber or wooden sandals) in areas of family or public use, such as home bathrooms or community showers and pools.

■ ■ ⓆⓊEST: Quickly and Accurate Assess the Patient Using SCHOLAR MAC

QuEST SCHOLAR is an acronym used to assess a patient to determine self-care candidate status and to identify which treatment would be most appropriate. See Chapter 1 for a description of the QuEST SCHOLAR process.

■ Does the Patient Have a Tinea Infection?

■ Inflammatory pattern at the edge of the lesion with varying degrees of redness and scaling or, occasionally, blister or vesicular formation

■ Lesions often have a clear center (ununiformed inflammatory response over the entire lesion) surrounded by an inflammatory edge.

■ Lesions may cause itching and pain.

■ Does the Patient Have Tinea Pedis (Feet)?

■ Fissuring, scaling, or maceration in the interdigital spaces of toes; malodor; pruritus; a stinging sensation on the feet; or combinations thereof.

■ Other variants may present with papules and scales with mild inflammation and diffuse hyperkeratotic dry scaling on the soles of the feet; presence of small vesicles or vesicopustules near the instep and on the midanterior plantar surface.

■ Does the Patient Have Tinea Corporis (Body)?

■ Circular, erythematous, pruritic, scaly lesions on any part of the body

■ Lesions are spread peripherally, and borders may contain vesicles or pustules.

■ Does the Patient Have Tinea Cruris (Groin)?

■ Tinea cruris occurs on the medial and upper parts of the thighs and the pubic area. In males, the lesions usually spare the penis and scrotum.

■ Lesions have well-demarcated margins that are elevated slightly and are more erythematous than the central area; small vesicles may be present, especially at the margins.

■ Acute lesions are bright red, and chronic cases tend to be more hyperpigmented.

■ Generally bilateral with scaling and significant pruritus

- See Table 1 for clinical presentation of other common dermatological disorders. These should be considered in the patient assessment.

Important SCHOLAR-MAC Considerations

- Where is/are the lesion(s) located?
    - Tinea infections of the scalp or nails are not self-treatable.

- Is the skin soggy or wet?
    - Wet, soggy types of tinea infections will also need treatment with aluminum salts in addition to topical antifungals.

- Are there other concurrent symptoms and characteristics?
    - Concurrent symptoms, such as purulent or excessive discharge, fever, or malaise, exclude the patient from self-treatment.

Physical Assessment Techniques

- Visually inspect the affected area if privacy and sanitary conditions allow.

TABLE 1. Differentiation of fungal skin infections and skin disorders with similar presentation

Criterion	Fungal Skin Infections	Contact Dermatitis	Bacterial Skin Infection
Location	On areas of the body where excess moisture accumulates, such as the feet, groin area, scalp, and under the arms	Any area of the body exposed to the allergen or irritant; hands, face, legs, ears, eyes, and anogenital area are most often involved	Anywhere on the body
Signs	Presents either as soggy, malodorous, thickened skin; acute vesicular rash; or fine scaling of affected area with varying degrees of inflammation; cracks and fissures may also be present	Presents as a variety of lesions: raised wheals, fluid-filled vesicles, or both	Presents as a variety of lesions from macules to pustules to ulcers with redness surrounding the lesion; lesions are often warmer than the surrounding unaffected skin
Symptoms	Itching and pain	Itching and pain	Irritation and pain
Quantity and severity	Usually localized to a single region of the body but can spread	Affects all areas of exposed skin but does not spread	Usually localized to a single region of the body but can spread
Timing	Variable onset	Variable onset from immediately after exposure to 3 weeks after contact	Variable onset
Cause	Superficial fungal infection	Exposure to skin irritants or allergens	Superficial bacterial infection
Modifying factors	Treated with nonprescription astringents, antifungals, and nondrug measures to keep the area clean and dry	Treated with topical antipruritics, skin protectants, astringents, and nondrug measures to avoid reexposure	Treated with prescription antibiotics

◼ ◼ QuⒺST: Establish that the patient is an appropriate self-care candidate

Utilize the information collected in the patient assessment with the treatment algorithm and exclusions for self-care to determine if self-care is appropriate.

◼ Exclusions to Self-Care

Review the treatment algorithm and exclusions for self-care provided at the beginning of the chapter. This section highlights key exclusion criteria.

◼ Medications

- Immune system suppressants (e.g., glucocorticoids) — the resulting impaired wound healing can decrease potential treatment option efficacy or require extended treatment duration beyond what is indicated for self-care.

◼ Conditions

- Patients with impaired wound healing or immune systems (e.g., diabetes, immune deficiency) or systemic infections are at a higher risk for development of tinea infections and should have their underlying conditions evaluated prior to self-treatment.

- Recurrent skin infections may be a sign of undiagnosed diabetes, immunodeficiency, or a circulatory problem that requires medical evaluation.

◼ Special Populations

- Pregnant patients should be treated by a primary care provider or OB/GYN.

◼ ◼ QuⒺⓈT: Suggest appropriate self-care strategies

Select the appropriate treatment option based on the previously collected patient data. Various treatment options are discussed along with clinical pearls and pertinent patient considerations for optimal management.

◼ Treatment Options

Tinea pedis, corporis, and cruris treatment of choice is topical antifungals.

■ Topical Antifungals

- Terbinafine and butenafine have the shortest length of treatment, with the ability to cure tinea pedis in 1 week. However, complete resolution of symptoms may require up to 4 weeks of treatment.
- Butenafine's effectiveness on infection of the bottom or sides of the foot is unknown; it may be most beneficial for tinea pedis between the toes.
- Tolnaftate is beneficial primarily in treating infections with dry, scaly lesions and is the only antifungal approved for both prevention and treatment of tinea infections.
- Clioquinol and undecylenic acid are approved for tinea pedis and cruris. These products are less effective on scalp or nails, despite commercial advertisement.
- Adverse effects may include skin irritation, burning, stinging, itching, and dryness.

CAUTIONS FOR TOPICAL ANTIFUNGALS

- A drug-drug interaction between warfarin and topical miconazole cream may increase the effects of warfarin.
- Delayed hypersensitivity reactions to tolnaftate may occur but are extremely rare.

Other Treatment Considerations

Wet, soggy type infection treatment of choice is salts of aluminum followed by topical antifungals.

- Solutions of 20% aluminum acetate and 20% aluminum chloride demonstrate equal in vitro antibacterial efficacy, which may help prevent secondary bacterial infections.
- Adverse effects associated with aluminum salts include irritation.

CAUTIONS FOR SALTS OF ALUMINUM

- Use on severely eroded or deeply fissured skin is contraindicated.
- Prolonged or continuous use of aluminum acetate solution may produce tissue necrosis—solution should not be used for more than 1 week.

- Complementary Therapy
  - Bitter orange, tea tree oil, and ajoene (a constituent of garlic believed to have antifungal activity) have been used with mixed success in the management of fungal skin infections, with few or no adverse effects. However, since none of the studies that examined these ingredients included more than 60 patients, the results of each complementary therapy warrant further investigation.

Special Populations

- Pregnancy
  - Pregnant patients should be treated by a primary care provider or OB/GYN.
  - Topical clotrimazole and miconazole are compatible during pregnancy and are FDA Pregnancy Risk Category B, but use during the first trimester should be avoided because of increased risk of spontaneous abortions (SABs). Although the risk for SABs was found in a study looking at vaginitis treatment, until there are more data, the application of these antifungals to large areas of the skin should also be avoided.[2]
  - Butenafine is considered Pregnancy Risk Category C in all trimesters.
  - Fetal risk for pregnancy cannot be ruled out for tolnaftate.
- Breastfeeding
  - Evidence for all nonprescription topical antifungals are inconclusive for determining infant risk when used during breastfeeding.

⬛⬛ QuES❶: Talk with the patient

Patient Education/Counseling

- Nonpharmacologic Talking Points
  - To prevent the spread of infection to other parts of the body, either use a separate towel to dry the affected area or dry the affected area last.
  - Do not share towels, clothing, or other personal articles with household members, especially when an infection is present.
  - Launder contaminated towels and clothing in hot water and dry them on a hot dryer setting to prevent the spread of infection.
  - Cleanse skin daily with soap and water and thoroughly pat dry to remove oils and other substances that promote growth of fungi.

- If possible, do not wear clothing or shoes that cause the skin to stay wet.
- If needed, allow shoes to dry thoroughly before wearing them again. Dust shoes with medicated or nonmedicated foot powder to help keep them dry.
- Avoid contact with people who have fungal infections. Wear protective footwear (e.g., rubber or wooden sandals) in areas of family or public use, such as home bathrooms or community showers.

- Pharmacologic Talking Points
  - Topical Antifungals
    - Creams or solutions are the most efficient and effective dosage forms for delivery of the active ingredient to the epidermis.
    - Proper application technique (apply a thin layer) for topical antifungals should be described.
    - Stress importance of completing the length of recommended therapy, even if symptoms resolve before the end of therapy.
  - Salts of Aluminum
    - For wet, soggy type or if oozing lesions are present, apply or soak area in aluminum acetate solution (1:40) before applying the antifungal.

- Suggest medical referral if any of the following occur:
  - The infection worsens, does not improve within a week, or persists beyond the recommended length of therapy

Clinical Pearls

- All topical antifungals for treating tinea infections are effective if used for the recommended length of therapy; the factors that influence selection of a specific agent will primarily depend on patient factors, such as adherence and dosage form preference.

- Products with similar brand names may differ in their active ingredients, depending on the dosage formulation. It is important to read the active ingredient on the Drug Facts label to confirm that the intended active ingredient is selected.

- The effectiveness of topical antifungals will be limited unless the patient follows nonpharmacological recommendations to eliminate other predisposing factors to tinea infections. Nonpharmacological measures will also prevent the spread of the infection to other parts of the body and other people.

■ ■ References

1. Gardner A, Walkup N. Fungal skin infections. In: Krinsky DL, Ferreri SP, Henstreet BA, Hume AL, Newton GD, Rollins CJ, Tietze KJ, eds. *Handbook of Nonprescription Drugs: An Interactive Approach to Self-Care.* Washington, DC: American Pharmacists Association; 2017:793–808.

2. Briggs GG, Freeman RK, eds. *Drugs in Pregnancy and Lactation: A Reference Guide to Fetal and Neonatal Risk.* 10th ed. Philadelphia, PA: Wolters Kluwer/Lippincott Williams & Wilkins Health; 2015.

HEADACHE

Connie Kang, PharmD, BCPS, BCGP

For complete information about this topic, consult Chapter 5, "Headache," written by Julie J. Wilkinson and Katherine Tromp and published in the *Handbook of Nonprescription Drugs*, 19th Edition.[1]

Self-Care of Headache

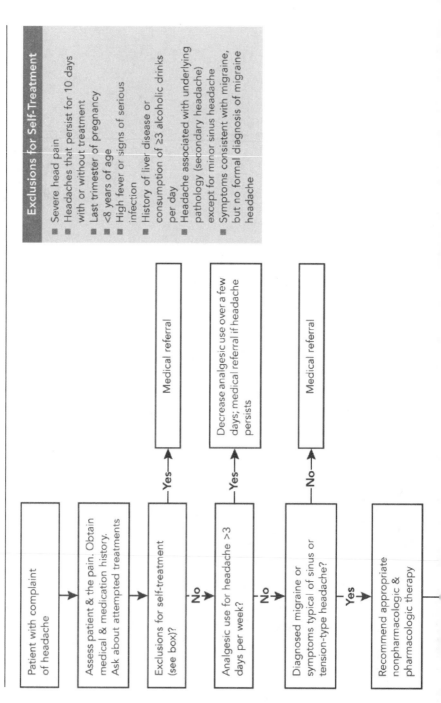

Exclusions for Self-Treatment

- Severe head pain
- Headaches that persist for 10 days with or without treatment
- Last trimester of pregnancy
- <8 years of age
- High fever or signs of serious infection
- History of liver disease or consumption of ≥3 alcoholic drinks per day
- Headache associated with underlying pathology (secondary headache) except for minor sinus headache
- Symptoms consistent with migraine, but no formal diagnosis of migraine headache

Patient with complaint of headache
↓
Assess patient & the pain. Obtain medical & medication history. Ask about attempted treatments
↓
Exclusions for self-treatment (see box)? —Yes→ Medical referral
↓ No
Analgesic use for headache >3 days per week? —Yes→ Decrease analgesic use over a few days; medical referral if headache persists
↓ No
Diagnosed migraine or symptoms typical of sinus or tension-type headache? —No→ Medical referral
↓ Yes
Recommend appropriate nonpharmacologic & pharmacologic therapy

(continued)

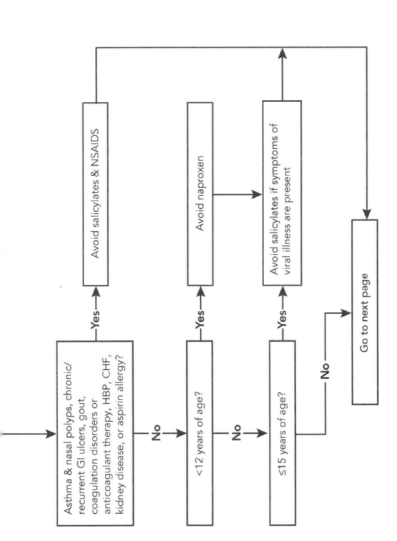

Asthma & nasal polyps, chronic/recurrent GI ulcers, gout, coagulation disorders or anticoagulant therapy, HBP, CHF, kidney disease, or aspirin allergy?

Yes → Avoid salicylates & NSAIDS

No

<12 years of age?

Yes → Avoid naproxen

No

≤15 years of age?

Yes → Avoid salicylates if symptoms of viral illness are present

No → Go to next page

Self-Care of Headache *(Continued)*

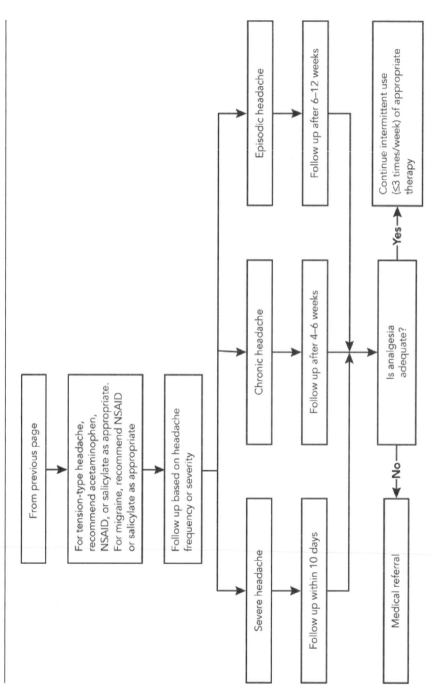

From previous page

For tension-type headache, recommend acetaminophen, NSAID, or salicylate as appropriate. For migraine, recommend NSAID or salicylate as appropriate

Follow up based on headache frequency or severity

Severe headache → Follow up within 10 days

Chronic headache → Follow up after 4–6 weeks

Episodic headache → Follow up after 6–12 weeks

Is analgesia adequate?

—No→ Medical referral

—Yes→ Continue intermittent use (≤3 times/week) of appropriate therapy

CHF = congestive heart failure; GI = gastrointestinal; HBP = high blood pressure; NSAID = nonsteroidal anti-inflammatory drug.

⬛⬤ Overview

- *Primary* headaches are not associated with an underlying medical condition; examples that are amendable to self-treatment include episodic and diagnosed chronic tension-type headaches, diagnosed migraine with and without aura, and medication-overuse headaches.

- *Secondary* headaches are symptomatic of an underlying physiologic condition; examples include head trauma, stroke, substance abuse or withdrawal, bacterial and viral diseases, and disorders of craniofacial structures. Secondary headaches other than minor sinus headaches are excluded from self-treatment.

- The goal of self-treatment is to relieve headache pain, prevent headaches when possible, and prevent medication-overuse headaches through avoiding chronic use of nonprescription analgesics.

⬛⬤ Pathophysiology

- *Tension-type headaches* often manifest in response to stress, anxiety, depression, emotional conflicts, and other stimuli. Episodic tension-type headaches are thought to result in pain felt by the peripheral nervous system, whereas chronic tension-type headaches are thought to result from stimuli to the central nervous system (CNS).

- *Migraine headaches* likely arise from a complex interaction of neuronal and vascular factors. Evidence suggests migraines occur through dysfunction of the trigeminovascular system. Migraine triggers may include bodily stressors, environmental factors, hormones, and medications.

- *Medication-overuse headaches* result from excessive use of analgesics, which is thought to cause a change from episodic headaches to chronic headaches. Medication-overuse headaches occur as a "rebound phenomenon" after repeated and excessive use of analgesics for episodic headache disorder.

- *Sinus headaches* occur when infection or blockage of the paranasal sinuses causes inflammation or distention of the sensitive sinus walls. Sinus congestion may be caused by viral infection, bacterial infection, or allergic rhinitis.

◼ Preventative Measures

◼ *Migraine headache* prevention includes avoiding personal triggers and observing the following general nutritional strategies:

- Eat regularly to avoid hunger and low blood sugar.
- Avoid foods or food additives with vasoactive substances known to trigger migraines: nitrites (e.g., cured meats), monosodium glutamate (e.g., Asian food), tyramine (e.g., aged cheese and red wine), phenylalanine (e.g., aspartame), caffeine, and theobromines (e.g., chocolate).
- Avoid personal food allergens.
- When onset of migraine headache is predictable, take an analgesic for migraine prevention:
  - Take two days before headache is expected and continue regular use throughout the time the headache might occur (e.g., menstrual migraine during menstruation).

◼ *Medication-overuse headache* prevention includes monitoring use of nonprescription analgesics:

- Do not use nonprescription analgesics more than 3 days per week to prevent medication-overuse headaches.

◼ ◼ QuEST: Quickly and Accurate Assess the Patient Using SCHOLAR MAC

QuEST SCHOLAR is an acronym used to assess a patient to determine self-care candidate status and to identify which treatment would be most appropriate. See Chapter 1 for a description of the QuEST SCHOLAR process.

◼ Does the Patient Have a Tension-Type Headache?

◼ The severity and duration of pain are highly variable.

◼ The pain initially feels like pressure or tightening on both sides of the head and subsequently may spread to feel like a band around the head.

◼ Duration of episodic tension-type headaches range from a few hours to several days:

- Episodic tension-type headaches occur less than 15 days per month.
- Chronic tension-type headaches 15 days or more per month for at least 3 months.

TABLE 1. Characteristics of tension-type, migraine, and sinus headaches

Feature	Tension-Type Headache	Migraine Headache	Sinus Headache
Location	Bilateral; over the top of the head, extending to neck	Usually unilateral	Face, forehead, or periorbital area
Nature	Varies from diffuse ache to tight, pressing, constricting pain	Throbbing; may be preceded by an aura	Pressure behind eyes or face; dull, bilateral pain
Onset	Gradual	Sudden	Simultaneous with sinus symptoms, including purulent nasal discharge
Duration	Hours to days	Hours to 2–3 days	Days (resolves with sinus symptoms)
Nonheadache symptoms	Scalp tenderness, neck pain and muscle tension	Nausea, vomiting	Nasal congestion

■ The major defining characteristics of tension-type, migraine, and sinus headaches are available in Table 1.

Does the Patient Have a Migraine Headache?

■ Patients may experience aura but can also have migraines without aura. Aura is a series of neurologic symptoms (e.g., "blind spots," shimmering or flashing in vision, visual or auditory hallucinations, muscle weakness).

■ Aura may last up to 30 minutes, and unilateral throbbing headache pain that follows may last from several hours to days.

■ Additional symptoms may include nausea, vomiting, photophobia, phono-phobia, tinnitus, light-headedness, vertigo, irritability, and sinus symptoms.

Does the Patient Have a Medication-Overuse Headache?

■ Patients who use analgesics more than 2–3 times weekly for 3 months or longer and experience headaches 15 or more days per month may experience medication-overuse headaches.

■ Headache frequency or severity may worsen over the period of medication overuse.

■ Patients may experience a nearly continuous headache, particularly on awakening. Additional symptoms patients may experience are difficulty concentrating, lethargy, irritability, and nausea.

■ Onset of the headache occurs within hours of stopping the agent, and readministration of the agent provides relief.

■ Does the Patient Have a Sinus Headache?

- ■ Usually localized to facial areas over the sinuses, can be difficult to differentiate from migraine without aura

- ■ Blowing the nose or bending down often intensifies the pain.

■ Important SCHOLAR MAC Considerations

- ■ Do the headaches seem to be associated with any exposure(s) or event(s) (e.g., food, stress)?

- ■ What does your headache feel like?
    - ▪ This can help determine which type of headache the patient is experiencing to determine if self-treatment is appropriate and optimal nonprescription treatments.

- ■ What have you tried to relieve the headache?
    - ▪ May help identify medication-overuse headache

■ ■ QuⒺST: Establish that the patient is an appropriate self-care candidate

Utilize the information collected in the patient assessment with the treatment algorithm and exclusions for self-care to determine if self-care is appropriate.

■ Exclusions to Self-Care

Review the treatment algorithm and exclusions for self-care provided at the beginning of the chapter. This section highlights key exclusion criteria.

■ Medications

- ■ Prescription and nonprescription analgesics—potential treatment options may be duplicative and risk serious adverse effects. A thorough assessment of a patient's medication history is needed, including combination analgesics.
    - ▪ If medication history includes use of nonprescription analgesics, caffeine, prescription, triptans, opioids, butalbital, or ergotamines, consider medication-overuse headache.

- If medication history includes oral contraceptives, postmenopausal hormones, nitrates, or reserpine, consider migraine.

- Antihypertensives—potential treatment options can raise blood pressure and counteract the mechanism of the antihypertensive (nonsteroidal anti-inflammatory drugs [NSAIDs] and angiotensin-converting enzyme [ACE] inhibitors). This is likely not clinically significant for short-term use, but patients should be warned of potential impact on blood pressure.

- Selective serotonin reuptake inhibitors (SSRI), selective norepinephrine reuptake inhibitors (SNRI), and monoamine oxidase inhibitors (MAOI)—potential use with decongestants for sinus headache can result in tachycardia.

- See Table 2 for a list of common drug interactions.

Conditions

- Cardiovascular diseases (e.g., heart failure, high blood pressure, previous heart attack) can be worsened by NSAID use. Short-term use for headache symptoms is likely okay.

- NSAIDs should be used cautiously in patients with renal dysfunction or conditions prone to renal dysfunction (e.g., diabetes).

- Acetaminophen should be used cautiously in patients with hepatic dysfunction or with a history of alcoholism or chronic alcohol abuse.

- A medical diagnosis of migraine headache is required before self-treatment is appropriate for migraines.

Special Populations

- Frail older adults may not be appropriate candidates for self-care; all non-prescription medications should be considered for appropriateness and dose adjustments made as needed.

- Patients in their last trimester of pregnancy should be cautiously treated after their OB/GYN has determined self-treatment is appropriate, as headache is a hallmark symptom of pre-eclampsia.

- Aspirin-containing products should not be used in children less than 16 years of age with viral illnesses because of the risk of Reye's syndrome.

TABLE 2. Clinically important drug-drug interactions with nonprescription analgesic agents

Analgesic, Antipyretic	Drug	Potential Interaction	Management and Preventive Measures
Acetaminophen	Alcohol	Increased risk of hepatotoxicity	Avoid concurrent use if possible; minimize alcohol intake when using acetaminophen.
Acetaminophen	Warfarin	Increased risk of bleeding (elevations in INR)	Limit acetaminophen to occasional use; monitor INR for several weeks when acetaminophen 2–4 g daily is added or discontinued in patients on warfarin.
Aspirin	Valproic acid	Displacement from protein-binding sites and inhibition of valproic acid metabolism	Avoid concurrent use; use naproxen instead of aspirin (no interaction).
Aspirin	NSAIDs, including COX-2 inhibitors	Increased risk of gastroduodenal ulcers and bleeding	Avoid concurrent use if possible.
Ibuprofen	Aspirin	Decreased antiplatelet effect of aspirin	Aspirin should be taken at least 30 minutes before or 8 hours after ibuprofen. Use acetaminophen (or other analgesic) instead of ibuprofen.
Ibuprofen	Phenytoin	Displacement from protein-binding sites	Monitor free phenytoin levels; adjust dose as indicated.
NSAIDs	Bisphosphonates	Increased risk of GI or esophageal ulceration	Use caution with concomitant use.
NSAIDs	Digoxin	Renal clearance of digoxin inhibited	Monitor digoxin levels; adjust dose as indicated.
Salicylates and NSAIDs	Antihypertensive agents, beta blockers, ACE inhibitors, vasodilators, diuretics	Antihypertensive effect inhibited; possible hyperkalemia with potassium-sparing diuretics and ACE inhibitors	Monitor blood pressure, cardiac function, and potassium levels.
Salicylates and NSAIDs	Anticoagulants	Increased risk of bleeding, especially GI	Avoid concurrent use if possible; risk is lowest with salsalate and choline magnesium trisalicylate.
Salicylates and NSAIDs	Alcohol	Increased risk of GI bleeding	Avoid concurrent use if possible; minimize alcohol intake when using salicylates and NSAIDs.
Salicylates and NSAIDs	Methotrexate	Decreased methotrexate clearance	Avoid salicylates and NSAIDs with high-dose methotrexate therapy; monitor levels with concurrent treatment.
Salicylates (moderate-high doses)	Sulfonylureas	Increased risk of hypoglycemia	Avoid concurrent use if possible; monitor blood glucose levels when changing salicylate dose.

Abbreviations used: ACE, Angiotensin-converting enzyme; COX, cyclooxygenase; INR, international normalized ratio; NSAID, nonsteroidal anti-inflammatory drug.

■ ● QuE⑤T: Suggest appropriate self-care strategies

Select the appropriate treatment option based on previously collected patient data. Various treatment options are discussed along with clinical pearls and pertinent patient considerations for optimal management.

● Treatment Options

Tension-type headache treatment of choice is a systemic analgesic.

■ Systemic Analgesics
- Nonprescription analgesics are usually effective in relieving tension-type headaches, especially when taken at the onset of the headache.
  - All nonprescription analgesics have an equivalent onset of action of 30 minutes, with varying durations of activity:
    - Acetaminophen lasts 4–6 hours.
    - Ibuprofen lasts 6–8 hours.
    - Naproxen lasts up to 12 hours.
- Generally, patients will desire rapid pain relief; thus, immediate release dosage forms should be recommended over extended release dosage forms.
- While acetaminophen does not have anti-inflammatory benefits, limited research supports that acetaminophen and ibuprofen should be considered equally effective for headaches.
- Individual patients may report a better response to one NSAID. As such, it may be effective to recommend an alternative NSAID when patients have previously failed to get relief from an NSAID.
- Aspirin is considered a superior analgesic versus nonacetylated salicylates (e.g., magnesium salicylate).
- Avoid NSAIDs in patients with aspirin intolerance; acetaminophen and nonacetylated salicylates (e.g., magnesium salicylate) are considered safe.
- Adverse effects associated with acetaminophen include nausea, hepatotoxicity, and skin rash (rare). It is well-tolerated when recommended doses are not exceeded.
- Adverse effects associated with NSAIDs include heartburn, dyspepsia, anorexia, epigastric pain, bleeding and bruising, and increased blood pressure.
- Adverse effects associated with salicylates include nausea, vomiting, bleeding, and dyspepsia.

CAUTIONS FOR ACETAMINOPHEN

- Acetaminophen is potentially hepatotoxic in doses exceeding 4 g/day, especially with chronic use.
- The FDA recommends an acetaminophen maximum daily dosage of 3000–3250 mg to lower the risk of accidental acetaminophen overdose.
- More conservative dosing (≤2 g/day) or avoidance may be considered in the following patients at increased risk for acetaminophen-induced hepatotoxicity: liver disease, 3 or more alcoholic drinks/day, concurrent hepatotoxic drug(s), and poor nutritional intake.

CAUTIONS FOR NSAIDs

- NSAIDs are associated with increased serious gastrointestinal (GI; e.g., ulceration, bleeding), cardiovascular (e.g., myocardial infarction, stroke, heart failure, uncontrolled high blood pressure), and nephropathy risks.
- Naproxen is considered the safer NSAID option for cardiovascular risk. Patients should take the minimum dose for the shortest duration to control symptoms.
- NSAID GI risk factors include age greater than 60 years, consuming 3 or more alcoholic drinks/day, previous ulcer disease in the case of GI bleeding, concurrent use of anticoagulants (including aspirin), and higher dose or longer duration of treatment.

CAUTIONS FOR SALICYLATES

- Avoid aspirin in patients with risk factors for upper GI bleeding. Risk factors include age greater than 60 years, 3 or more alcoholic drinks/day, history of peptic ulcer, and concomitant use of NSAIDs, anticoagulants, antiplatelet agents, bisphosphonates, SSRIs, or systemic corticosteroids.
- Avoid use of aspirin-containing products with uncontrolled high blood pressure, heart failure, bleeding disorders, or renal failure.
- Avoid effervescent aspirin solutions with high sodium content in patients who have hypertension, heart failure, or renal failure.

Migraine headache treatment of choice is NSAIDs.

- NSAIDs
  - Both ibuprofen and naproxen can be considered. Both agents have an onset of approximately 30 minutes; duration is 6–8 hours for ibuprofen and up to 12 hours for naproxen.
  - Analgesics work best at the early stages of a migraine; taking an NSAID at the onset of symptoms can abort a mild or moderate migraine headache.
  - Individual patients may report a better response to one NSAID. As such, it may be effective to recommend an alternative NSAID when patients have previously failed to get relief from an NSAID.
  - Avoid NSAIDs in patients with aspirin intolerance; acetaminophen and nonacetylated salicylates (e.g., magnesium salicylate) are considered safe.
  - Adverse effects associated with NSAIDs include heartburn, dyspepsia, anorexia, epigastric pain, bleeding and bruising, and increased blood pressure.

> **CAUTIONS FOR NSAIDs**
> - NSAIDs are associated with increased serious GI (e.g., ulceration, bleeding), cardiovascular (e.g., myocardial infarction, stroke, heart failure, uncontrolled high blood pressure), and nephropathy risks.
> - Naproxen is considered the safer NSAID option for cardiovascular risk. Patients should take the minimum dose for the shortest duration to control symptoms.
> - NSAID GI risk factors include age greater than 60 years, 3 or more alcoholic drinks/day, previous ulcer disease in the case of GI bleeding, concurrent use of anticoagulants (including aspirin), and higher dose or longer duration of treatment.

- Salicylates
  - Aspirin may be considered for use for migraine treatment, but generally risks outweigh benefits at the dose required for anti-inflammatory effects.
    - Doses required for anti-inflammatory effects (4–6 g/day) are at or exceed the maximum nonprescription dose (4 g/day) and are substantially higher than required NSAID doses for anti-inflammatory effects.

- For patients requiring rapid pain relief, enteric-coated aspirin is inappropriate because of the delay in absorption and prolonged onset of analgesic effect.
- Adverse effects associated with salicylates include nausea, vomiting, bleeding, and dyspepsia.

CAUTIONS FOR SALICYLATES

- Avoid aspirin in patients with risk factors for upper GI bleeding. Risk factors include age greater than 60 years, 3 or more alcoholic drinks/day, history of peptic ulcer, and concomitant use of NSAIDs, anticoagulants, antiplatelet agents, bisphosphonates, SSRIs, or systemic corticosteroids.
- Avoid use of aspirin-containing products with uncontrolled high blood pressure, heart failure, bleeding disorders, or renal failure.
- Avoid effervescent aspirin solutions with high sodium content in patients who have hypertension, heart failure, or renal failure.

Medication-overuse headache treatment of choice is tapering and eliminating the offending agent(s).

- Patient may decrease analgesic use over a few days. May need to refer to primary care if headache persists for prescription therapy for headaches during the days to weeks of the withdrawal period.

Sinus headache treatments of choice are oral or topical decongestants (e.g., pseudoephedrine, oxymetazoline) with a nonprescription analgesic.

- Oral Decongestants
    - Pseudoephedrine is the oral decongestant of choice; efficacy of phenylephrine has been highly debated.
    - Adverse effects associated with decongestants include cardiovascular stimulation (e.g., elevated blood pressure, tachycardia, palpitation, arrhythmias) and CNS stimulation (e.g., restlessness, insomnia, anxiety, tremors, fear, hallucinations).

CAUTIONS FOR ORAL DECONGESTANTS

- Patients with hypertension should use systemic decongestants only with medical advice.

- Decongestants are contraindicated in patients receiving concomitant MAOIs and for 2 weeks after discontinuation.
- Persons taking an SSRI or SNRI antidepressant should use decongestants with caution, as these medications may increase heart rate.

- Topical Decongestants
  - Topical decongestants may be preferred over oral decongestants in patients with comorbidities.
  - Adverse effects associated with topical decongestants are primarily administration-related because of minimal systemic absorption and include propellant- or vehicle-associated effects (e.g., burning, sneezing, local dryness).

  CAUTIONS FOR TOPICAL DECONGESTANTS
  - Patients with hypertension should use topical decongestants cautiously.

- Systemic Analgesics
  - Acetaminophen or NSAIDs (naproxen, ibuprofen) can be used with a decongestant to provide additional pain relief from congestion caused by a sinus headache.
  - Avoid NSAIDs in patients with aspirin intolerance; acetaminophen and nonacetylated salicylates (e.g., magnesium salicylate) are considered safe.
  - Adverse effects associated with acetaminophen include nausea, hepatotoxicity, and skin rash (rare). It is well-tolerated when recommended doses are not exceeded.
  - Adverse effects associated with oral NSAIDs include heartburn, dyspepsia, anorexia, epigastric pain, bleeding and bruising, and increased blood pressure.

  CAUTIONS FOR ACETAMINOPHEN
  - Acetaminophen is potentially hepatotoxic in doses exceeding 4 g/day, especially with chronic use.
  - The FDA recommends an acetaminophen maximum daily dosage of 3000–3250 mg to lower the risk of accidental acetaminophen overdose.

- More conservative dosing (≤2 g/day) or avoidance may be considered in the following patients at increased risk for acetaminophen-induced hepatotoxicity: liver disease, 3 or more alcoholic drinks/day, concurrent hepatotoxic drug(s), and poor nutritional intake.

CAUTIONS FOR NSAIDs

- NSAIDs are associated with increased serious GI (e.g., ulceration, bleeding), cardiovascular (e.g., myocardial infarction, stroke, heart failure, uncontrolled high blood pressure), and nephropathy risks.
- Naproxen is considered the safer NSAID option for cardiovascular risk. Patients should take the minimum dose for the shortest duration to control symptoms.
- NSAID GI risk factors include age greater than 60 years, 3 or more alcoholic drinks/day, previous ulcer disease in the case of GI bleeding, concurrent use of anticoagulants (including aspirin), and higher dose or longer duration of treatment.

Other Treatment Considerations

- Avoid combination products with caffeine and nonprescription analgesics, as caffeine may trigger migraines and caffeine withdrawal may cause headache.

- Combination of NSAIDs, aspirin, and/or acetaminophen may achieve goals of pain relief with lower doses of the individual agents. However, insufficient evidence is available to support the safety and effectiveness of this practice.

- Complementary Therapy
- Butterbur, feverfew, and coenzyme Q10 are commonly used for the prevention of migraine headaches. Use should be avoided in pregnancy and lactation.
  - Butterbur is considered effective for the prevention of migraine by both the American Academy of Neurology and the American Headache Society, including some positive results in children and adolescents.
    - Use products labeled as pyrrolizidine alkaloid–free.
    - Use a butterbur dose of 50–75 mg twice daily for 4–6 months and then taper to the lowest tolerated dose without return of migraines.
    - The maximum duration of use for which safety has been established is 12–16 weeks.

- Feverfew leaf is considered probably effective for the prevention of migraine by the American Academy of Neurology and the American Headache Society, but long-term safety and efficacy have not been established.
    - Use a feverfew dose of 50–100 mg/day in divided doses or 6.25 mg CO_2 standardized extract (MIG-99) 2–3 times daily.
    - Do not stop taking abruptly, as postfeverfew syndrome may result in anxiety, headaches, insomnia, and muscle stiffness from withdrawal.
- Coenzyme Q10 dose for migraine prevention is 100 mg/day for children and 300 mg/day for adults.

- Other unproven remedies include peppermint oil applied to the forehead and temples for treatment of tension headaches and magnesium for treatment and prevention of migraine headaches.

Special Populations

Pregnancy

- Acetaminophen has long been considered safe in pregnancy, but emerging evidence suggests there may be a slight association between maternal prenatal use of acetaminophen and attention deficit hyperactivity disorder (ADHD) in the child. Duration of use that is less than 8 days is negatively associated with ADHD. Duration of use that is more than 29 days has the greatest association. Patients should be advised of this potential association; however, short-term use appears nonsignificant.[2]
- Limit NSAID use to clinical situations in which the potential benefit justifies potential fetal risk because of potential complications with delivery (e.g., prolonged labor, increased postpartum bleeding) and harm to fetus (e.g., premature closing of the ductus arteriosus); NSAIDs are contraindicated in the third trimester.
- Avoid aspirin during pregnancy, especially during the last trimester, because of risk of maternal and fetal harm.
- Avoid oral decongestants during pregnancy because of theoretical decreased fetal blood flow. Oxymetazoline is the preferred topical decongestant during pregnancy because of poor absorption.

Breastfeeding

- Acetaminophen appears in breast milk but is considered compatible with breastfeeding. A rarely occurring maculopapular rash in infants, which subsides with discontinuation, is the only adverse effect reported in infants exposed through breast milk.

- Naproxen should be avoided in nursing mothers. It is unknown whether ibuprofen is excreted in human milk. Thus, ibuprofen use should be carefully weighed against potential harm to the infant.
- Avoid aspirin during breastfeeding because of potential risk of adverse platelet function in nursing infants.
- The American Academy of Pediatrics (AAP) has found pseudoephedrine compatible with breastfeeding. Because decongestants may decrease milk production, lactating mothers should monitor their milk production and drink extra fluids as needed.
- Topical oxymetazoline and phenylephrine are considered "probably compatible" in breastfeeding women because of a lack of available human data. Therefore, pseudoephedrine is the preferred decongestant in breastfeeding mothers.

■ Pediatric Patients
- For children less than 12 years of age, preference is to dose acetaminophen and ibuprofen based on body weight, rather than age, using the table provided on the product.
- Naproxen is not indicated for children less than 12 years of age.
- Topical decongestants may be preferred over oral decongestants in children greater than 8 years of age with sinus headaches.

■ Geriatric Patients
- Acetaminophen is generally recognized as the agent of choice for mild-moderate pain in the geriatric population because of the increased risk of serious GI, hypertensive, and renal effects of NSAIDs and salicylates.
- Topical decongestants may be preferred over oral decongestants in older adults with sinus headaches.

■ ■ QuES⬤: Talk with the patient

⬤ Patient Education/Counseling

■ Nonpharmacologic Talking Points
- Identification and strategies to decrease triggers should be discussed to help improve headache frequency.

- For chronic tension-type headaches, stretching and strengthening of head and neck muscles may be beneficial.
- Cold packs applied with pressure to the forehead or temple areas may provide relief for acute migraine pain.
- Encourage patients with frequent episodes to log triggers, frequency, intensity, duration of episodes, and response to treatment.
  - This can help the patient prevent headaches and assist the health care provider in optimizing treatment selection.

- Pharmacologic Talking Points
  - Systemic Analgesics
    - Do not delay nonprescription analgesic therapy. Outcomes are optimized by treating early in the course of the headache.
    - Do not use nonprescription analgesics more than 3 days per week to prevent medication-overuse headache.
    - Oral dosage forms are preferred over rectal because of slow and unreliable rectal absorption; however, rectal dosage forms may be preferred for patients experiencing migraine headache with severe nausea.
    - Completely chew chewable tablets, then drink a full glass of water.
    - NSAIDs and salicylates should be taken with food or milk to decrease GI irritation.
    - Patients should be reminded of the maximum dosages of non-prescription analgesic treatment:
      - Ibuprofen maximum dose is 1200 mg/day.
      - Naproxen sodium maximum dose is 660 mg/day.
      - Acetaminophen maximum dose is 3000–3250 mg/day.
  - Systemic Decongestants
    - Avoid decongestant use near bedtime because of adverse effects of insomnia and restlessness.
    - Advise to monitor for adverse effects (e.g., elevated blood pressure, elevated blood glucose) in patients with conditions sensitive to adrenergic stimulation (e.g., hypertension, diabetes).
    - The maximum dose of pseudoephedrine is 240 mg daily.
  - Topical Decongestants
    - The patient should not use topical decongestants longer than 3–5 days because of risk for rebound congestion.

■ Suggest medical referral if any of the following occur:
  ▪ Headaches persist longer than 3 days or worsen despite self-treatment.
  ▪ Experience chronic tension-type headache
  ▪ Patients with diagnosed migraine headaches are not adequately self-treated
  ▪ Chronic congestion and sinus infections, as it may be a sign of structural abnormalities
  ▪ Signs and symptoms of a bacterial infection develop (e.g., oral temperature >101.5°F [38.0°C], significant ear pain, chest congestion, wheezing)

▣ Clinical Pearls

■ Use of a single oral analgesic is preferred over combination products that combine NSAIDs, aspirin, or acetaminophen, based on safety and effectiveness.

■ Treat the initiating headache type first to abort the mixed headache in patients with coexisting tension and migraine headaches.

■ Acetaminophen 1000 mg appears to have equivalent pain relief properties to naproxen 375 mg for episodic tension-type headache.

■ Naproxen sodium 220 mg and ibuprofen 200 mg appear to have similar efficacy.

▣▣ References

1. Wilkinson JJ, Tromp K. Headache. In: Krinsky DL, Ferreri SP, Hemstreet BA, Hume AL, Newton GD, Rollins CJ, Tietze KJ, eds. *Handbook of Nonprescription Drugs: An Interactive Approach to Self-Care.* Washington, DC: American Pharmacists Association; 2017:77–96.

2. Ystrom E, Gustavson K, Brandlistuen RE, et al. Prenatal exposure to acetaminophen and risk of ADHD. *Pediatrics.* 2017;140(5):e20163840.

▣▣ Additional References

1. Lemay V, Feret B. Fever. In: Krinsky DL, Ferreri SP, Hemstreet BA, Hume AL, Newton GD, Rollins CJ, Tietze KJ, eds. *Handbook of Nonprescription Drugs: An Interactive Approach to Self-Care.* Washington, DC: American Pharmacists Association; 2017:97–110.

2. Scolaro K. Colds and allergy. In: Krinsky DL, Ferreri SP, Hemstreet BA, Hume AL, Newton GD, Rollins CJ, Tietze KJ, eds. *Handbook of Nonprescription Drugs: An Interactive Approach to Self-Care*. Washington, DC: American Pharmacists Association; 2017:189–216.

3. McQueen CE, Orr KK. Natural products. In: Krinsky DL, Ferreri SP, Hemstreet BA, Hume AL, Newton GD, Rollins CJ, Tietze KJ. *Handbook of Nonprescription Drugs: An Interactive Approach to Self-Care*. Washington, DC: American Pharmacists Association; 2017:957–994.

HEARTBURN

Jennifer A. Wilson, PharmD, BCACP
and Rashi Chandra Waghel, PharmD, BCACP

For complete information about this topic, consult Chapter 13, "Heartburn and Dyspepsia," written by Tara Whetsel and Ann Zweber and published in the *Handbook of Nonprescription Drugs*, 19th Edition.[1]

Self-Care of Heartburn

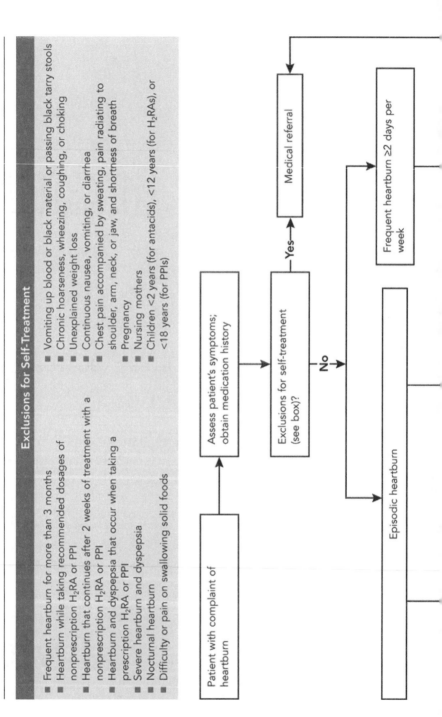

Exclusions for Self-Treatment

- Frequent heartburn for more than 3 months
- Heartburn while taking recommended dosages of nonprescription H$_2$RA or PPI
- Heartburn that continues after 2 weeks of treatment with a nonprescription H$_2$RA or PPI
- Heartburn and dyspepsia that occur when taking a prescription H$_2$RA or PPI
- Severe heartburn and dyspepsia
- Nocturnal heartburn
- Difficulty or pain on swallowing solid foods
- Vomiting up blood or black material or passing black tarry stools
- Chronic hoarseness, wheezing, coughing, or choking
- Unexplained weight loss
- Continuous nausea, vomiting, or diarrhea
- Chest pain accompanied by sweating, pain radiating to shoulder, arm, neck, or jaw, and shortness of breath
- Pregnancy
- Nursing mothers
- Children <2 years (for antacids), <12 years (for H$_2$RAs), or <18 years (for PPIs)

Patient with complaint of heartburn

Assess patient's symptoms; obtain medication history

Exclusions for self-treatment (see box)?

Yes → Medical referral

No →

Episodic heartburn

Frequent heartburn ≥2 days per week

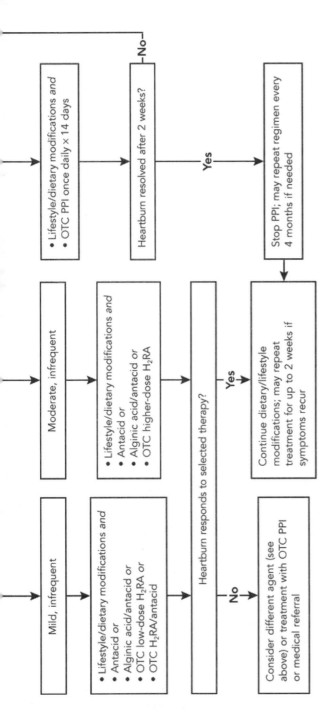

H₂RA = histamine H₂-receptor antagonist; OTC = over-the-counter; PPI = proton pump inhibitor.

◼️◼️ Overview

- Heartburn is a common gastrointestinal (GI) issue and is often described as a burning sensation that starts in the stomach or lower chest and moves upward.

- Heartburn is most often mild and episodic; however, it can occur on a more frequent basis (≥2 days per week). Heartburn is a common symptom of gastroesophageal reflux disease (GERD).

- Dyspepsia is discomfort in the upper abdomen that is characterized by epigastric pain, burning, postprandial fullness, early satiety, or combinations thereof.

- Goals for self-treatment of heartburn and dyspepsia include resolution of symptoms, reduced recurrence of symptoms, and prevention and management of medication adverse effects.

◼️◼️ Pathophysiology

- The lower esophageal sphincter (LES) prevents the stomach contents from traveling back up into the esophagus. However, transient relaxation of the LES can result in reflux of gastric acid. This can lead to esophageal tissue damage over time. Heartburn can also be stimulated by certain foods or beverages that trigger sensory nerve endings in the esophagus, resulting in reflux of gastric acid.

- The pathophysiology of dyspepsia is not well-defined and can be associated with factors similar to heartburn.

- See Table 1 for risk factors that may contribute to heartburn and dyspepsia. T1

◼️◼️ QuEST: Quickly and Accurate Assess the Patient Using SCHOLAR MAC

QuEST SCHOLAR is an acronym used to assess a patient to determine self-care candidate status and to identify which treatment would be most appropriate. See Chapter 1 for a description of the QuEST SCHOLAR process.

◼️ Does the Patient Have Heartburn or Dyspepsia?

- Heartburn usually appears as a burning sensation behind the breastbone that moves upward from the chest within an hour of eating, especially if the meal is large or contains trigger foods or beverages. Symptoms can occur at night, interfering with sleep (nocturnal heartburn).

TABLE 1. Risk factors that may contribute to heartburn and dyspepsia

Dietary	Medications
Alcohol (ethanol)	Alpha-adrenergic antagonists
Caffeinated beverages	Anticholinergic agents
Carbonated beverages	Aspirin, NSAIDs
Chocolate	Barbiturates
Citrus fruit or juices	Benzodiazepines
Coffee	Beta-2 adrenergic agonists
Fatty foods	Bisphosphonates
Garlic or onions	Calcium channel blockers
Mint (e.g., spearmint, peppermint)	Chemotherapy
Salt and salt substitutes	Clindamycin
Spicy foods	Dopamine
Tomatoes or tomato juice	Doxycycline
	Estrogen
Lifestyle	Iron
Exercise (isometric, running)	Narcotic analgesics
Obesity	Nitrates
Smoking (tobacco)	Potassium
Stress	Progesterone
Supine body position	Prostaglandins
Tight-fitting clothing	Quinidine
	TCAs
Diseases	Tetracycline
Motility disorders (e.g., gastroparesis)	Theophylline
PUD	Zidovudine
Scleroderma	
Zollinger-Ellison syndrome	**Other**
	Genetics
	Pregnancy

Abbreviations used: PUD, peptic ulcer disease; NSAID, nonsteroidal anti-inflammatory drug; TCA, tricyclic antidepressant.

■ Dyspepsia includes postprandial fullness, early satiation, epigastric pain, or burning. Other less specific symptoms may include bloating, nausea, vomiting, and belching.

Important SCHOLAR MAC Considerations

■ How often and how long has the patient experienced symptoms?
  ■ Treatment options depend on the frequency and severity of symptoms.
    □ Episodic or infrequent heartburn occurs less than 2 days per week.
      – It can be mild (a little bothersome and does not interfere with normal activities) or moderate (somewhat bothersome, interferes with normal activities, or both).

       ▫ Frequent heartburn occurs 2 or more days per week.
- If frequent heartburn is persistent (lasting 3 or more months), GERD may be suspected, which is an exclusion for self-treatment.

- Is the patient experiencing any alarm symptoms or atypical or extraesophageal symptoms?
  - Alarm symptoms can indicate more severe disease, complications, or both, which require medical referral. These include dysphagia (difficulty swallowing), odynophagia (painful swallowing), upper GI bleeding, and unexplained weight loss.
  - Some patients may exhibit atypical or extraesophageal symptoms, including noncardiac chest pain, difficulty breathing, hoarseness, laryngitis, chronic cough, dental erosion, or feeling of a lump in the throat. These patients also require medical referral.

■ ■ QuⒺST: Establish that the patient is an appropriate self-care candidate

Utilize the information collected in the patient assessment with the treatment algorithm and exclusions for self-care to determine if self-care is appropriate.

■ Exclusions to Self-Care

Review the treatment algorithm and exclusions for self-care provided at the beginning of the chapter. This section highlights key exclusion criteria.

■ Medications

- Certain antifungals and antivirals may interact with histamine-2 receptor antagonists (H2RAs) and proton pump inhibitors (PPIs).

- Cimetidine is associated with more drug interactions than other H2Ras, since it inhibits several cytochrome P450 (CYP) enzymes, which can limit its use.

- PPIs inhibit CYP2C9, which can increase the concentration of drugs that are metabolized through this enzyme.

- Omeprazole and esomeprazole may inhibit certain variants of CYP2C19, leading to less conversion of clopidogrel to its active form, resulting in a reduced antiplatelet effect.

- See Table 2 for a summary of drug interactions involving antacids, H2RAs, and PPIs and preventative and management strategies.

Conditions

- Caution should be used with using aluminum- or magnesium-containing antacids in patients with poor renal function. If H2RAs are used, they should be at lower doses.

- Sodium bicarbonate antacids should be avoided in patients taking cardio-vascular medications because of an increased risk of fluid overload.

TABLE 2. Clinically important drug-drug interactions with nonprescription heartburn and dyspepsia agents

Drug	Effect	Management and Preventative Measures
Drug Interactions Caused by Alterations in Intragastric pH		
Atazanavir, indinavir, iron supplements, itraconazole, ketoconazole	Decreased absorption of these drugs	Separate from antacids by at least 2 hours Avoid concurrent use of H2RAs and PPIs or closely monitor
Enteric-coated products	Premature breakdown of enteric coating	Separate from antacids by at least 2 hours
Drugs That May Interact with Antacids		
Azithromycin, fluoroquinolones, tetracyclines	Decreased absorption of these drugs	Separate from antacids by at least 2 hours for azithromycin, 4 hours for tetracyclines, and 6 hours for fluoroquinolones
Isoniazid	Decreased absorption when administered with aluminum hydroxide	Take isoniazid at least 1 hour prior
Salicylates	Increased urinary excretion and decreased blood concentration of these drugs	Avoid concurrent use of salicylates and sodium bicarbonate or closely monitor
Amphetamines, quinidine	Increased blood concentration of these drugs	Separate amphetamines from antacids by at least 2 hours. Avoid concurrent use of quinidine and sodium bicarbonate or closely monitor
Drugs That May Interact with Cimetidine		
Amiodarone, phenytoin, theophylline, tricyclic antidepressants, warfarin, clopidogrel	Cimetidine inhibits CYP450 3A4, 2D6, 1A2, and 2C9.	Avoid concurrent use.
Drugs That May Interact with PPIs		
Cilostazol	Increased blood concentration of cilostazol	Avoid concurrent use; lansoprazole may be a safer alternative.
Clopidogrel	Esomeprazole and omeprazole reduces antiplatelet effect	Avoid concurrent use.
Diazepam, phenytoin, tacrolimus, theophylline, warfarin	Increased blood concentrations of these drugs (CYP2C19 inhibition)	Avoid concurrent use.
Methotrexate	Increased risk of methotrexate toxicity	Avoid concurrent use of high-dose methotrexate

- Constipating antacids (e.g., calcium or aluminum) should be avoided in patients prone to constipation, while diarrhea-causing antacids (e.g., magnesium) should be avoided in patients prone to diarrhea.

● Special Populations

- There are no products available for children less than 2 years of age for the treatment of heartburn or dyspepsia.

- Pregnant women experiencing frequent or moderate-severe heartburn should receive medical referral.

- Older adults with new-onset heartburn or dyspepsia should receive special consideration. These patients are more likely to be taking medications that can cause heartburn. They may also be at increased risk of having a more severe underlying condition or complications from heartburn.

● ● QuE⑤T: Suggest appropriate self-care strategies

Select the appropriate treatment option based on the previously collected patient data. Various treatment options are discussed along with clinical pearls and pertinent patient considerations for optimal management.

● Treatment Options

Mild-to-moderate episodic or infrequent heartburn treatments of choice include antacids, H2RAs, or a combination of both.

- Antacids
    - Antacids have a generally quick onset (<5 minutes). They have a short duration of action (20–30 minutes), but it is slightly prolonged in the presence of food.
    - Alginic acid, often listed as an inactive ingredient, is sometimes added to provide a protective barrier to reduce esophageal irritation.
    - Adverse effects vary and depend on the active ingredient, but antacids are generally well-tolerated.
        - Magnesium-containing antacids are associated with dose-related diarrhea.
        - Calcium-containing antacids may cause belching and flatulence as well as constipation.

◦ Aluminum-containing antacids more commonly cause dose-related constipation but can also cause hypophosphatemia with excessive use.

◦ Sodium bicarbonate antacids often result in belching and flatulence.

CAUTIONS FOR ANTACIDS

- Magnesium-containing antacids should not be used in impaired renal function (creatinine clearance [CrCl] < 30 mL/min).
- Patients taking calcium-containing antacids should be mindful of concomitant agents containing calcium.
- Chronic use of aluminum-containing antacids should be avoided in patients with renal failure.
- Sodium bicarbonate antacids may cause fluid overload and therefore should be used cautiously in those with congestive heart failure, renal failure, cirrhosis, pregnancy, and sodium-restricted diets.

- Histamine-2 Receptor Antagonists
  - H2RAs are preferred over antacids in patients with mild-to-moderate episodic heartburn who require more prolonged relief or when antacids are insufficient.
  - The onset of action is 30–45 minutes with a duration of 4–10 hours.
  - H2RAs can be used in combination with antacids when both quick relief and an extended duration of action is required.
  - At the recommended doses, there are only minor differences in potency, onset, duration, and adverse effects.
  - Adverse effects include headache, diarrhea, constipation, dizziness, and drowsiness. Cimetidine can be associated with additional anti-androgenic adverse effects at higher doses.

CAUTIONS FOR H2RAs

- A dose reduction should be considered for patients of advanced age, impaired renal function, or both (CrCl < 50 mL/min).

Frequent heartburn treatments of choice are PPIs or H2RAs.

- Proton Pump Inhibitors (PPIs)
  - PPIs are not intended for immediate relief of occasional or acute episodes.

- The onset of action is 2–3 hours with a duration of 12–24 hours. Complete relief can take 1–4 days.
- Differences in efficacy among available PPIs have not been established.
- Adverse effects include diarrhea, constipation, and headache.

CAUTIONS FOR PPIs

- PPI tablets and capsules should not be chewed or crushed, as that may affect the release and effectiveness of the medication.
- Chronic use (in excess of the recommended nonprescription dosing) is associated with an increased risk for adverse effects, such as infections, fractures in older adult patients, chronic kidney disease, dementia, vitamin B_{12} deficiency, hypomagnesemia, and iron malabsorption. Many of these adverse effects occur when use exceeds one year, which is much greater than the nonprescription approved dosing.

Other Treatment Considerations

- Bismuth Subsalicylate
  - Bismuth subsalicylate (BSS) can be used for heartburn, upset stomach, indigestion, nausea, and diarrhea.
  - Adverse effects include dark-colored stools and tongue.

CAUTIONS FOR BSS

- Patients allergic to aspirin should not use BSS.
- BSS is approved for patients 16 years of age and older. Reye's syndrome is rare but can occur.
- If a patient is taking aspirin or other salicylate-containing drugs, toxic levels of salicylate may be reached even if the patient follows dosing directions on the label for each medication.
- BSS is not recommended in pregnant or nursing women or patients with bleeding risk.

- Complementary Therapy
  - There is no current evidence that any natural products relieve heartburn by increasing stomach pH.
  - Both peppermint and artichoke leaf extract have been shown to help with dyspepsia symptoms.

■ Special Populations

■ Pregnancy

- Lifestyle modifications are first-line in pregnancy. If these measures are insufficient for treating infrequent or mild heartburn in pregnancy, calcium- and magnesium-containing products can be used safely as long as the recommended daily intake is not exceeded.
- H2RAs are generally considered safe in pregnancy and may be considered if lifestyle modifications and antacids are insufficient.
- Medical referral should be recommended for pregnant patients with frequent or moderate-severe heartburn. If PPIs are appropriate, lansoprazole and omeprazole have the most safety evidence in pregnancy.

■ Breastfeeding

- Aluminum-, calcium-, or magnesium-containing acids are considered safe in women who are breastfeeding.
- H2RAs are compatible with breastfeeding, with famotidine being the preferred agent.
- PPIs should be avoided during breastfeeding, as there is insufficient evidence to support use.

■ Pediatric Patients

- Calcium-containing antacids can be used in children 2 years of age and older for mild, transient, and infrequent heartburn.
- H2RAs are approved for use in patients 12 years and older.
- PPIs are approved for use in patients 18 years and older.

■ Geriatric Patients

- Older adult patients are often on multiple medications, some of which can contribute to heartburn or dyspepsia and are provided in Table 1. They are also at a higher risk for developing complications or having a more severe underlying condition.
- Antacids can be used in older adult patients with no specific contraindications. When selecting an agent, consideration may be given to whether or not the patient is predisposed to either constipation or diarrhea.
- When using H2RAs, lower doses should be used in older adult patients, particularly if they are at increased risk for delirium according to the Beers List for Potentially Inappropriate Use of Medications in Older

Adults. Cimetidine should be avoided because of the increased risk of adverse effects and drug interactions.[2]

- *PPIs were added to the Beers List in 2015* because of *an association between PPI exposure and infections, bone loss, and fractures.*[2]

▦ ▦ QuES❶: Talk with the patient

▦ *Patient Education/Counseling*

■ Nonpharmacologic Talking Points
   - Lifestyle modifications should be recommended for all patients. These measures are aimed at avoidance of triggers and reduction of esophageal acid exposure.
   - Patients can monitor their diet and lifestyle to help identify triggers.
   - Medications should be evaluated to determine if they are contributing to heartburn symptoms.
   - Weight loss is recommended in overweight or obese patients to help relieve heartburn symptoms.
   - Patients should eat smaller meals, reduce dietary fat intake, and avoid eating within 3 hours of lying down.
   - Patients should abstain from or limit use of tobacco products, alcohol, and caffeine.
   - Avoid tight-fitting clothing, as this can exacerbate heartburn symptoms.
   - If lying down after eating cannot be avoided, a foam wedge can be used or the head of the bed can be elevated with blocks to help reduce symptoms.

■ Pharmacologic Talking Points
   - Antacids
      □ These agents should be administered at the onset of symptoms, and relief should generally be expected within 5 minutes. Liquid formulations may have a slightly quicker onset of action. These medications do not have a very long duration of action, though it is increased in the presence of food.
      □ Generally, antacids should not be used more than 4 times daily.
      □ Diarrhea may occur with magnesium-containing antacids, whereas constipation may occur with calcium- or aluminum-containing antacids.

- H2RAs
  - These agents can be administered at onset of symptoms or 30–60 minutes prior to anticipated symptoms. Relief should be expected within 30–45 minutes. H2RAs should be administered on an as-needed basis.
  - These agents should not be used more than 2 times daily for greater than 2 weeks.
  - It is recommended administration be as needed rather than on a scheduled basis to avoid tolerance.
  - H2RA in combination with an antacid may provide quicker relief than an H2RA alone and more sustained relief than an antacid alone.
  - Lower doses of H2RAs are best for mild, infrequent heartburn, while higher doses should be reserved for moderate, infrequent symptoms.
- PPIs
  - PPIs should be dosed daily, 30–60 minutes before a meal, ideally breakfast. Complete resolution should occur within 4 days of treatment initiation.
  - Self-care should be limited to 14 days, no more than once every 4 months.
  - Patients should not crush or chew tablets or capsules.
- BSS
  - Patients should be made aware that BSS can cause the stool or tongue to turn black.
  - BSS can be given every 30–60 minutes as needed and is not to exceed 4 doses in 24 hours.

- Suggest medical referral if any of the following occur:
  - Heartburn or dyspepsia continues after 2 weeks of continuous treatment with a nonprescription medication at recommended doses
  - Heartburn or dyspepsia lasts for more than 3 months
  - Heartburn awakens the patient during the night
  - Alarm symptoms (e.g., dysphagia, unexplained weight loss, upper GI bleeding)
  - Atypical or extraesophageal symptoms (e.g., chest pain, asthma, chronic cough)
  - Continuous nausea, vomiting, diarrhea, or severe stomach pain

● *Clinical Pearls*

■ Self-treatment of heartburn and dyspepsia should be limited to mild or moderate symptoms. Product selection will depend on patient specific factors (e.g., symptom frequency and severity, concomitant medications, comorbid conditions, product formulation preferences, product cost).

■ Patients should review product labels carefully to ensure that they remain within daily recommended intake or dosages.

■ Healthcare providers should screen patients for use of a prescription H2RA or PPI and counsel patients to avoid duplication of therapies.

● ● References

1. Whetsel T and Zweber A. Heartburn and dyspepsia. In: Krinsky DL, Ferreri SP, Henstreet BA, Hume AL, Newton GD, Rollins CJ, Tietze KJ, eds. *Handbook of Non-prescription Drugs: An Interactive Approach to Self-Care*. Washington, DC: American Pharmacists Association; 2017:233–250.

2. American Geriatrics Society 2015 Beers Criteria Update Expert Panel. American Geriatrics Society 2015 updated Beers Criteria for potentially inappropriate medication use in older adults. *J Am Geriatr Soc*. 2015 Nov;63(11):2227–2246.

INSOMNIA

Albert Bach, PharmD

For complete information about this topic, consult Chapter 46, "Insomnia, Drowsiness, and Fatigue," written by Sarah T. Melton and Cynthia K. Kirkwood and published in the *Handbook of Nonprescription Drugs*, 19th Edition.[1]

Self-Care of Transient and Short-Term Insomnia

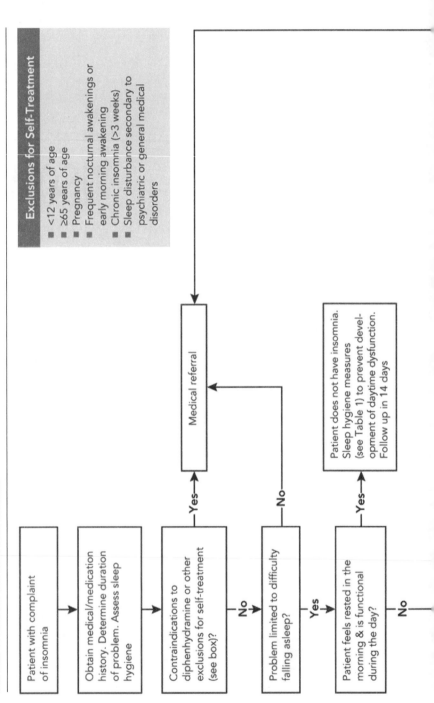

Exclusions for Self-Treatment

- <12 years of age
- ≥65 years of age
- Pregnancy
- Frequent nocturnal awakenings or early morning awakening
- Chronic insomnia (>3 weeks)
- Sleep disturbance secondary to psychiatric or general medical disorders

Patient with complaint of insomnia

↓

Obtain medical/medication history. Determine duration of problem. Assess sleep hygiene

↓

Contraindications to diphenhydramine or other exclusions for self-treatment (see box)? — **Yes** → Medical referral

↓ **No**

Problem limited to difficulty falling asleep? — **No** → Medical referral

↓ **Yes**

Patient feels rested in the morning & is functional during the day? — **Yes** → Patient does not have insomnia. Sleep hygiene measures (see Table 1) to prevent development of daytime dysfunction. Follow up in 14 days

↓ **No**

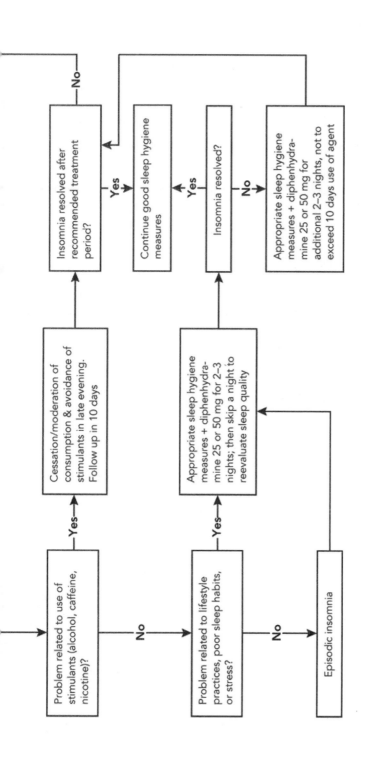

■ ■ Overview

- Insomnia occurs when a person has trouble falling or staying asleep, wakes up early and cannot return to sleep, or does not feel refreshed after sleeping, and this impaired sleep interferes with daytime function.

- The majority of U.S. adults experience insomnia a few nights a week, with the typical adult getting only 6.7 hours out of the required 8+ hours of sleep nightly.

- The goal of treating insomnia is to normalize sleep patterns to improve the patient's sleep quality and quantity and improve daytime functioning.

■ ■ Pathophysiology

- There is no universally accepted model for the nature, etiology, and pathophysiology of insomnia, but various models have contributed insomnia to physiologic hyperarousal in both central and peripheral nervous systems, genetics, endogenous sleep-promoting or wake-suppressing substances, and electrophysiologic and physiologic dysregulation in the wake and sleep brain network.[2]

- Insomnia can be classified as follows:
    - Transient insomnia: less than 1 week
    - Short-term insomnia: 1–3 weeks
    - Chronic or long-term insomnia: 3 weeks to years

■ Causes

- Acute life stresses (e.g., divorce, death of a loved one) or medical illness (e.g., depression, pain, gastroesophageal reflux disease [GERD]), anxiety, and poor sleep habits

- Travel, hospitalization, or anticipation of an important or stressful event can cause transient insomnia.

- Shift workers often complain of sleep disturbances, excessive sleepiness, or both.

- Stimulant effects of caffeine, nicotine, or other medications

- Late-night exercise and late-evening meals

- Environmental distractions, such as noise, lighting, uncomfortable temperatures, or new surroundings

- Alcohol can cause insomnia after acute use and as a withdrawal effect after chronic use.

- Prescription and nonprescription medications can produce either insomnia or withdrawal insomnia. Medications known to cause insomnia are antidepressants, antihypertensive agents, and sympathomimetic amines, such as pseudoephedrine and phenylephrine.

● Preventative Measures

- Insomnia with no underlying medical cause can be prevented with good sleep hygiene practices. These practices involve a combination of cognitive therapy, sleep restriction, stimulus control, and behavioral interventions. A list of sleep hygiene measures is available in Table 1.

■ ■ QuEST: Quickly and Accurate Assess the Patient Using SCHOLAR MAC

QuEST SCHOLAR is an acronym used to assess a patient to determine self-care candidate status and to identify which treatment would be most appropriate. See Chapter 1 for a description of the QuEST SCHOLAR process.

● Does the Patient Have Insomnia?

- Complaints of difficulty falling asleep, frequent awakening, early morning awakening and inability to fall back to sleep, disturbed quality of sleep with unusual or troublesome dreams, or just poor sleep in general.

TABLE 1. Principles of good sleep hygiene

- Use bed for sleeping or intimacy only.
- Establish a regular sleep pattern. Go to bed and arise at about the same time daily, even on the weekends.
- Make the bedroom comfortable for sleeping. Avoid temperature extremes, noise, and light.
- Engage in relaxing activities before bedtime.
- Avoid using electronic devices (particularly videos, television, and tablets) around bedtime.
- Exercise regularly but not within 2–4 hours of bedtime.
- If hungry, eat a light snack, but avoid eating meals within 2 hours before bedtime.
- Avoid daytime napping.
- Avoid using caffeine, alcohol, or nicotine for at least 4–6 hours before bedtime.
- If unable to fall asleep, do not continue to try to sleep; rather, get out of bed and perform a relaxing activity until you feel tired.
- Do not watch the clock at night.

- Sleep impairment occurs despite adequate opportunity and conditions for sleep.

- Some impairment in daytime functioning, such as daytime fatigue, decreased concentration or motivation, or memory impairment, must also be reported for a diagnosis of insomnia.

◖ Important SCHOLAR MAC Considerations

- How long has the patient been experiencing insomnia?
    - Determine if it is transient, short-term, or chronic (long-term) insomnia.

- Does the patient use any stimulants (e.g., caffeine, nicotine)?

- Does the patient consume alcohol?
    - Alcohol can initially improve sleep, but sleep disturbances occur in the second half of the night at high doses.
    - Heavy and chronic alcohol drinkers usually experience restless sleep and reduced sleep duration. Chronic alcohol drinkers may also have an irregular or disorganized sleep cycle.

- Are there problems related to lifestyle practices, poor sleep habits, or stress?
    - First-line treatment of insomnia should incorporate correction of these problems through sleep hygiene.

◖ ◖ QuⒺST: Establish that the patient is an appropriate self-care candidate

Utilize the information collected in the patient assessment with the treatment algorithm and exclusions for self-care to determine if self-care is appropriate.

◖ Exclusions to Self-Care

Review the treatment algorithm and exclusions for self-care provided at the beginning of the chapter. This section highlights key exclusion criteria.

◖ Medications

- Patients with secondary insomnia caused by the use or withdrawal of medications should be referred to the patient's primary care provider to manage the medications.

■ Drugs that can cause insomnia include, but are not limited to, anabolic steroids, antidepressants (e.g., bupropion, fluoxetine, venlafaxine), clonidine, amphetamines, decongestants, beta blockers (especially propranolol), corticosteroids, nicotine, oral contraceptives, and thyroid preparations.

■ Drugs that can produce withdrawal insomnia include, but are not limited to, amphetamines, first-generation ("sedating") antihistamines, barbiturate, benzodiazepines, illicit drugs (e.g., cocaine, marijuana, phencyclidine), monoamine oxidase inhibitors (MAOIs), opiates, and tricyclic antidepressants.

■ Drugs with anticholinergic properties (e.g., first-generation [sedating] antihistamines, incontinence medications, tricyclic antidepressants [TCAs], etc.) — potential treatment option will have an additive anticholinergic burden, and, generally, these combinations should not be used together.

◼ Conditions

■ Chronic insomnia is often the result of underlying medical problems (e.g., sleep apnea, narcolepsy), psychiatric disorders, or substance abuse and will require medical referral.

■ Frequent nocturnal awakenings or early morning awakening may suggest circadian rhythm disorders or depression and should be considered for medical referral.

◼ Special Populations

■ Pregnant patients may not be appropriate candidates for self-care; safety of antihistamines during pregnancy has not been well established, and use should be discussed with the patient's obstetrician.

■ Diphenhydramine may cause paradoxical excitation in younger children, which may cause difficulty sleeping. Generally, it should be avoided for this reason.

■ The Beers Criteria recommend avoiding the use of anticholinergic drugs in older adults. Nonprescription first-generation (sedating) antihistamines should not be recommended in patients 65 years of age or older.

◼ ◼ QuEST: Suggest appropriate self-care strategies

Select the appropriate treatment option based on the previously collected patient data. Various treatment options are discussed along with clinical pearls and pertinent patient considerations for optimal management.

■ Treatment Options

Insomnia treatment of choice is first-generation (sedating) antihistamines.

■ First-Generation (Sedating) Antihistamines

- Diphenhydramine is the antihistamine of choice and the only FDA-approved nonprescription sleep aid deemed safe and effective for self-care.
- Tolerance to the sedative effect of diphenhydramine develops within days of repeated use, and therefore, patients should have an "off" night from diphenhydramine after 3 consecutive days of use to reduce tolerance.
- Doxylamine safety and efficacy as a sleep aid have not been fully established.
- Adverse effects associated with first-generation antihistamines may include dry mouth and throat, constipation, blurred vision, urinary retention, and tinnitus.

CAUTIONS FOR FIRST-GENERATION (SEDATING) ANTIHISTAMINES

- First-generation antihistamines are contraindicated in prostatic hyperplasia and angle-closure glaucoma.
- Children tend to be more sensitive to central nervous system (CNS) excitatory effects, while adults are more likely to experience CNS depression.
- First-generation antihistamines are listed as Potentially Inappropriate Medications for Older Adults in the 2015 American Geriatrics Society (AGS) Beers Criteria. The AGS recommends avoiding use in older adults. Use in patients with dementia may worsen cognitive decline.
- Patients with lower respiratory tract diseases (e.g., asthma, chronic obstructive pulmonary disease [COPD], chronic bronchitis) should use first-generation (sedating) antihistamines with caution, as they may mask signs and symptoms of worsening disease.
- Sedation from sleep aids may impair the ability to drive or operate machinery.
- Concomitant use with alcohol can have additive CNS depression and sedation.
- Diphenhydramine should not be used for long-term management of insomnia.

- Complementary Therapy
  - The American Academy of Sleep Medicine recommends against the use of dietary supplements to treat insomnia, unless approved by a health care provider.
  - Evidence of the effectiveness of melatonin for sleep disturbances in healthy people is inconclusive. Melatonin may have better responses in patients with developmental or neurologic disorders, elderly patients, depressed patients with sleep disorders, and those experiencing jet lag. The recommended dose of melatonin for insomnia is 0.3–5 mg taken 30 minutes prior to bedtime.
  - Valerian (*Valeriana officinalis*) at 400–900 mg of valerian root extract has limited benefit in insomnia compared with placebo. Continuous nightly use for several days or weeks is required for an effect, so valerian is not useful for acute insomnia. Patients using large dosages of valerian may experience severe benzodiazepine-like withdrawal symptoms and cardiac complications. Valerian should be slowly tapered after extended use.
  - Kava (*Piper methysticum*) use as a sleep aid has been associated with severe hepatotoxicity and therefore should be not recommended.

Special Populations

- Pregnancy
  - The safety of antihistamines during pregnancy has not been established, although most epidemiologic studies have not demonstrated increased risk of teratogenicity with the use of diphenhydramine during the first trimester. One trial did observe cleft palate alone and with other fetal abnormalities in children with first trimester exposures to diphenhydramine.
  - Behavioral interventions and good sleep hygiene are preferred treatment for insomnia in pregnancy.

- Breastfeeding
  - There is an increased risk of CNS adverse effects in breastfed infants following maternal intake of a sedating antihistamine. Therefore, it is recommended that nursing mothers use intermittent low dosages of diphenhydramine after the last daytime feeding to lessen potential adverse effects in the infant.

- Pediatric Patients
  - Diphenhydramine and doxylamine are not approved for insomnia in children under 12 years of age, and thus, they are not recommended for use in infants.

- Behavioral interventions and good sleep hygiene are first-line treatment for insomnia in children and adolescents.

- Geriatric Patients
  - Diphenhydramine and doxylamine can increase the risk of falls and cognitive and memory impairment in older adults and should not be recommended.
  - Recommend behavioral interventions and good sleep hygiene for older adults.

■ ■ QuESⓉ: Talk with the patient

● Patient Education/Counseling

- Nonpharmacologic Talking Points
  - Educate about sleep hygiene and encourage patients to implement strategies that are relevant for their nighttime activities.
  - See Table 1 for a detailed list of sleep hygiene practices.

- Pharmacologic Talking Points
  - First-Generation (Sedating) Antihistamines (Diphenhydramine)
    - Establish a regular bedtime routine and take diphenhydramine 30–60 minutes before the patient desires to go to sleep.
    - Do not take more than 50 mg of diphenhydramine each night.
    - Sedation from sleep aids may impair the ability to drive and operate machinery.
    - Taking nonprescription sleep aids can cause next-day sedation. To prevent next-day sedation, patients should ensure adequate time for sleep if taking a sleep aid.
    - After 2–3 nights of improved sleep, skip taking the medication for one night to see if the insomnia is relieved.
    - Do not self-treat for more than 10 consecutive nights.

- Suggest medical referral if any of the following occur:
  - Symptoms worsen or do not improve after 10 days

● Clinical Pearls

- Exploring the patient's behaviors and activities a few hours before bedtime, during bedtime, and upon awakening in the morning can reveal factors that may be contributing to or perpetuating the patient's insomnia. These factors should be addressed before starting drug therapy.

■ Many nonprescription combination products contain diphenhydramine as an active ingredient (e.g., Tylenol PM contains acetaminophen and diphenhydramine); health care providers should evaluate existing therapy and advise patients to avoid duplicate therapy or active ingredients that are not needed.

References

1. Melton ST, Kirkwood CK. Insomnia, drowsiness, and fatigue. In: Krinsky DL, Ferreri SP, Hemstreet BA, Hume AL, Newton GD, Rollins CJ, Tietze KJ, eds. *Handbook of Nonprescription Drugs: An Interactive Approach to Self-Care*. Washington, DC: American Pharmacists Association; 2017:855–872.

2. Levenson JC, Kay DB, Buysse DJ. The pathophysiology of insomnia. *Chest*. 2015;147(4):1179–1192.

3. McQueen CE and Orr KK. Natural products. In: Krinsky DL, Ferreri SP, Henstreet BA, Hume AL, Newton GD, Rollins CJ, Tietze KJ, eds. *Handbook of Nonprescription Drugs: An Interactive Approach to Self-Care*. Washington, DC: American Pharmacists Association; 2017:957–994.

4. American Geriatrics Society 2015 Beers Criteria Update Expert Panel. American Geriatrics Society 2015 Updated Beers Criteria for Potentially Inappropriate Medication Use in Older Adults. *J Am Geriatr Soc*. 2015 Nov;63(11):2227–2246.

MUSCULOSKELETAL INJURIES AND DISORDERS

Cortney M. Mospan, PharmD, BCACP, BCGP

For complete information about this topic, consult Chapter 7, "Musculoskeletal Injuries and Disorders," written by Julie L. Olenak and published in the *Handbook of Nonprescription Drugs*, 19th Edition.[1]

Self-Care of Musculoskeletal Injuries and Disorders

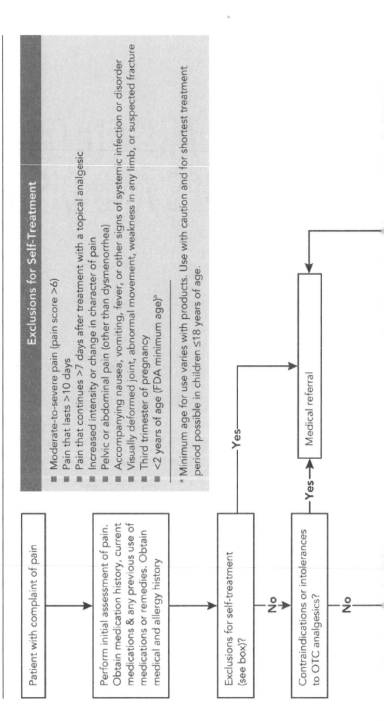

Exclusions for Self-Treatment

- Moderate-to-severe pain (pain score >6)
- Pain that lasts >10 days
- Pain that continues >7 days after treatment with a topical analgesic
- Increased intensity or change in character of pain
- Pelvic or abdominal pain (other than dysmenorrhea)
- Accompanying nausea, vomiting, fever, or other signs of systemic infection or disorder
- Visually deformed joint, abnormal movement, weakness in any limb, or suspected fracture
- Third trimester of pregnancy
- <2 years of age (FDA minimum age)[a]

[a] Minimum age for use varies with products. Use with caution and for shortest treatment period possible in children ≤18 years of age.

Patient with complaint of pain

Perform initial assessment of pain. Obtain medication history, current medications & any previous use of medications or remedies. Obtain medical and allergy history

Exclusions for self-treatment (see box)?

No → **Contraindications or intolerances to OTC analgesics?**

Yes → **Medical referral**

Yes → **Medical referral**

No

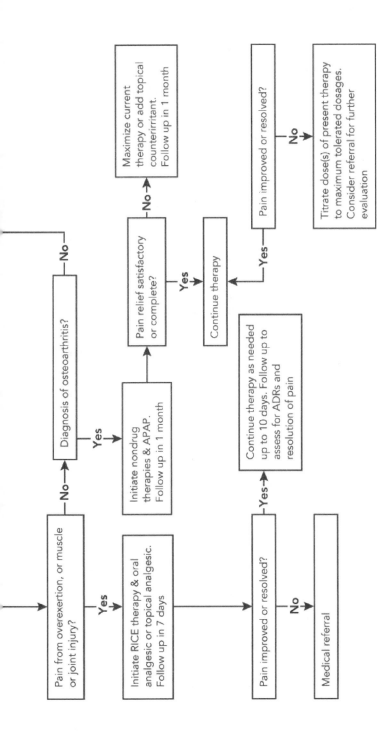

ADR = adverse drug reaction; APAP = acetaminophen; OTC = over-the-counter; RICE = rest, ice, compression, elevation.

■ ■ Overview

- Musculoskeletal pain arises from joints, bones, muscles, and connective tissue.

- Musculoskeletal pain may be felt in the affected tissue itself or referred from another anatomical location (e.g., hip pain caused by lower back injury).

- Pain can be acute (e.g., sports injuries), which lasts 4 weeks or less, or an exacerbation of a chronic, pathologic condition (e.g., osteoarthritis), which lasts longer than 3 months.

- Goals of therapy include decreasing pain duration and severity, restoring function, and preventing acute pain from progressing to chronic pain.

■ ■ Pathophysiology

- The musculoskeletal system includes the muscles, tendons, ligaments, cartilage, and bones. Because of high tensile strength, tendons and ligaments rarely rupture unless subjected to intense forces. They may become damaged when the joint is hyperextended or overused.

- Overuse or injury to the muscle, joint, or surrounding tissues causes stimulation of pain receptors located within skeletal muscle and overlying fascia.

- Erythema, edema, and hyperalgesia represent the inflammatory response.

■ ■ QuEST: Quickly and Accurate Assess the Patient Using SCHOLAR MAC

QuEST SCHOLAR is an acronym used to assess a patient to determine self-care candidate status and to identify which treatment would be most appropriate. See Chapter 1 for a description of the QuEST SCHOLAR process.

Table 1 provides a comparison of various musculoskeletal symptoms and T1 conditions.

■ Is the Patient Experiencing Lower Back Pain?

- Major risk factors for developing lower back pain include improper technique in lifting heavy objects, poor posture, improper shoes, excessive body

TABLE 1. Comparison of musculoskeletal disorders

	Myalgia	Tendonitis	Bursitis	Sprain	Strain	Osteoarthritis
Location	Muscles of the body	Tendon locations around joint areas	Inflammation of the bursae within joints; common locations include knee, shoulder, big toe	Stretching or tearing of a ligament within a joint	Hyperextension of a joint that results in overstretching or tearing the muscle or tendon	Weight-bearing joints, knees, hips, low back, hands
Signs	Possible swelling (rare)	Warmth, swelling, erythema	Warmth, edema, erythema, and possible crepitus	Swelling, bruising	Swelling, bruising	Noninflammatory joints, narrowing of joint space, restructuring of bone and cartilage (resulting in joint deformities), possible joint swelling
Symptoms	Dull, constant ache (sharp pain relatively rare); weakness and fatigue of muscles also common	Mild-severe pain generally occurring after use; loss of range of motion	Constant pain that worsens with movement or application of external pressure over the joint	Initial severe pain followed by pain, particularly with joint use; tenderness; reduction in joint stability and function	Initial severe pain with continued pain upon movement and at rest; muscle weakness; loss of some function	Dull joint pain relieved by rest; joint stiffness <20–30 minutes; localized symptoms to joint; crepitus
Onset	Varies depending on cause (e.g., trauma = acute, but drug-induced = insidious)	Often gradual, but can develop suddenly	Acute with injury; recurs with precipitant use of joint	Acute with injury	Acute with injury	Insidious development over years
Modifying Factors	Elimination of cause; use of stretching, rest, heat, topical analgesics; systemic analgesics	Elimination of cause; use of stretching, rest, ice, topical analgesics; systemic analgesics	Joint rest; immobilization; topical analgesics; systemic analgesics	RICE; stretching; use of protective wraps (e.g., ankle tape, knee brace, cane); topical analgesics; systemic analgesics	RICE; stretching; use of protective wraps; topical analgesics; systemic analgesics	Continuous exercise (light-moderate activity); weight loss, heat, analgesic medication; topical pain relievers

weight, poor mattress and sleeping postures, and sudden bursts of activity in an otherwise sedentary individual.

- Identifying the underlying cause for long-term symptom control and prevention is optimal.

- Most patients will recover in a few days or weeks, even without treatment.

Is the Patient Experiencing Overexertion?

- This is muscle damage that is typically initiated by force generated by muscle fibers when patients who were not previously physically active begin physical activity at a high level.

- Muscle soreness is the typical presenting symptom, typically with delayed onset (≥8 hours), which can last for days and generally peaks at 24–48 hours.

Is the Patient Experiencing Myalgia?

- Myalgia is muscle pain that presents as widespread or bilateral pain that is not typically associated with a recent injury.

- This can result from systemic infections, chronic disorders, medications, and alcohol abuse.

Does the Patient Have Bursitis?

- Bursitis is an inflammation of the bursa (fluid-filled sacs between joint spaces) that occurs from an acute joint injury or over-repetitive joint action. It presents with localized pain, swelling, and tenderness.

- Symptoms are worsened by movement of structures adjacent to bursa in the joint.

Does the Patient Have a Sprain?

- Sprains are damaged ligaments that are either overly stretched or torn.

- Sprains typically occur during physical activity.

- Sprains are graded by their characteristics, which determine their severity.

- Moderate-severe sprains should be referred for evaluation. Moderate-severe sprains present with significant pain, inability to bear weight, and loss of function in the affected limb(s).

Does the Patient Have a Strain?

- Strains are an injury to a muscle or tendon.

- Strains can occur from acute injury or prolonged overuse and can become chronic conditions.

- Strains typically occur from actions that involve twisting or pulling and when the capacity is exceeded (e.g., hyperextension).

Does the Patient Have Tendonitis?

- This is an inflammation of a tendon resulting from acute injury or chronic repetitive movements of a body part.

- Symptoms can present in many locations within the body: hand and wrist (carpal tunnel), Achilles tendon, etc.

- Certain medications (fluoroquinolones) are associated with the development of tendonitis or tendon rupture.

Does the Patient Have Osteoarthritis?

- Osteoarthritis is a degenerative joint disease. This condition is a gradual softening and destruction of the cartilage between bones.

- Repetitive movement, heavy physical activity, and lifting of heavy weights may aggravate the condition.

- Symptoms persist even without activity or when the joint is not in use, including during sleep.

- Pain level does not correlate with joint damage.

Important SCHOLAR MAC Considerations

- What is the pain quantity (pain score) and quality?
    - Inquiries should discuss cause, duration, severity, location, and factors that relieve or exacerbate pain.
    - Use of a pain scale can help quantify the intensity of a patient's pain. Patients can rank their pain on a numerical scale of 0–10 (0 being no pain, 10 being the worst imaginable pain).
    - In general, nonprescription medications are appropriate for scores of 1–3 and potentially 4 or 5. Scores of 6 or higher should be referred.

    - More extensive injuries (affecting a larger joint or multiple joints) will need oral analgesics.

- What is the patient's acceptable pain level?
    - Since pain is subjective, it is important to work with the patient to see an impact on that patient's pain score, realizing a score of 0 is likely not possible.

- What are the patient's activities of daily living?
    - Preventing reinjury and disability is a key goal of musculoskeletal injury treatment. Identifying a patient's activities of daily living and strategies to improve capacity for these can prevent further injury and damage.

Physical Assessment Techniques

- Observe the patient's joints and limbs for visible deformations; if present, emergency medical assistance should be sought.
- Observe the patient's injury for swelling, including gentle palpation of the injured area.
- Patients should be encouraged to be cautious with movement of the injured joint. If there is an apparent sprain associated with obvious limitations in joint function, the injury is likely a moderate or severe sprain. This will require proper workup by a health care provider to rule out a fracture or tear.

QuEST: Establish that the patient is an appropriate self-care candidate

Utilize the information collected in the patient assessment with the treatment algorithm and exclusions for self-care to determine if self-care is appropriate.

Exclusions to Self-Care

Review the treatment algorithm and exclusions for self-care provided at the beginning of the chapter. This section highlights key exclusion criteria.

Medications

- Prescription and nonprescription analgesics—potential treatment options may be duplicative and risk serious adverse effects. A thorough assessment of a patient's medication history is needed, including combination analgesics.

- Antihypertensives—potential treatment options can raise blood pressure and counteract the mechanism of the antihypertensive (nonsteroidal anti-inflammatory drugs [NSAIDs] and angiotensin-converting enzyme (ACE) inhibitors). This is likely not clinically significant for short-term use, but patients should be warned of long-term use of these therapies together.

- Table 2 provides a list of clinically important drug-drug interactions that should be considered.

Conditions

- Pain associated with osteoarthritis can only be managed with self-treatment after an initial medical diagnosis.

- When joint pain is accompanied by a puncture site, adjacent infection, or severe inflammation, infection should be ruled out before self-treatment is initiated.

TABLE 2. Clinically important drug-drug interactions with nonprescription analgesic agents

Analgesic	Potentially Interacting Drug	Potential Effect	Management and Preventive Measures
Acetaminophen	Alcohol	Increased risk of hepatotoxicity	Avoid concurrent use if possible; minimize alcohol intake when using acetaminophen.
Acetaminophen	Warfarin	Increased risk of bleeding (elevations in INR)	Limit acetaminophen to occasional use; most relevant with doses of ≥2 g/day of acetaminophen
Ibuprofen	Aspirin (cardiovascular prophylaxis)	Decreased antiplatelet effect of aspirin	Aspirin should be taken at least 30 minutes before or 8 hours after ibuprofen. Use acetaminophen (or other analgesic) instead of ibuprofen.
NSAIDs	Bisphosphonates	Increased risk of GI or esophageal ulceration	Use caution with concomitant use.
NSAIDs	Digoxin	Renal clearance of digoxin inhibited	Monitor digoxin levels; adjust dose as indicated.
Salicylates and NSAIDs	Antihypertensive agents, beta blockers, ACE inhibitors, vasodilators, diuretics	Antihypertensive effect inhibited; possible hyperkalemia with potassium-sparing diuretics and ACE inhibitors	Monitor blood pressure, cardiac function, and potassium levels.
NSAIDs	Anticoagulants	Increased risk of bleeding, especially GI	Avoid concurrent use, if possible.
NSAIDs	Alcohol	Increased risk of GI bleeding	Avoid concurrent use, if possible; minimize alcohol intake when using NSAIDs.
NSAIDs	Methotrexate	Decreased methotrexate clearance	Avoid NSAIDs with high-dose methotrexate therapy.

Abbreviations used: ACE, Angiotensin-converting enzyme; INR, international normalized ratio; NSAID, nonsteroidal anti-inflammatory drug.

- Chronic musculoskeletal conditions and immunologic conditions (e.g., rheumatoid arthritis, gout) use oral analgesics to manage these conditions. Medical history and current medications should be verified to avoid duplicative therapies.

■ Special Populations

- Pregnant patients should be referred to their primary care provider or OB/GYN to eliminate other causes and ensure medication safety.

- Pediatric patients 2 years of age or younger should be referred to their pediatrician.

- Older adults (≥75 years of age) should preferentially be recommended topical NSAIDs rather than oral NSAIDs because of the increased risk of adverse effects (e.g., acute kidney injury, cardiovascular events, gastrointestinal [GI] bleeds).

■ ■ QuE⑤T: Suggest appropriate self-care strategies

Select the appropriate treatment option based on the previously collected patient data. Various treatment options are discussed along with clinical pearls and pertinent patient considerations for optimal management.

■ Treatment Options

Lower back pain treatment of choice is NSAIDs.

- NSAIDs
    - NSAIDs should be first-line for acute lower back pain. NSAIDs have been found to provide some improvement in pain and function. NSAIDs should be recommended over acetaminophen if there is not a contraindication.
        - Topical NSAIDs can be used in patients when oral NSAIDs are contraindicated, but this is prescription only.
    - Acetaminophen should not be used for lower back pain, as it has been found to have no effect on pain and function.
    - Doses should be administered on a scheduled basis, starting as early as possible in the course of the injury. A quick tapering of dose and dosing interval should occur as the injury improves (typically 1–3 days).

- Chronic lower back pain first-line treatment is nonpharmacologic approaches.
- Adverse effects associated with oral NSAIDs include heartburn, dyspepsia, anorexia, epigastric pain, bleeding and bruising, and increased blood pressure.

> **CAUTIONS FOR NSAIDs**
>
> - Chronic use of NSAIDs can cause nephropathy, bleeding, increased cardiovascular events (e.g., myocardial infarction [MI], stroke, heart failure), and GI ulcerations, among other risks.
> - GI risks are greatest in patients who are 60 years of age and older, have a history of peptic ulcer disease, consume 3 or more alcoholic beverages/day, and use higher doses, longer duration of treatment, or both.
> - Risks may outweigh the benefits in patients 75 years and older; topical NSAIDs should be considered.

Mild-moderate aches and pains (tendonitis, bursitis, sprains, strains) treatment of choice is systemic analgesics.

- Systemic Analgesics
    - Acetaminophen and NSAIDs (ibuprofen, naproxen, magnesium salicylate, aspirin) are used in the initial treatment of musculoskeletal injuries.
    - These agents are considered to essentially be equivalent in terms of analgesic efficacy. Selection should be based on patient preferences, risk factors, current health conditions, and current medications (Table 2 provides relevant drug-drug interactions.)
    - Generally, acetaminophen is preferred in noninflammatory diseases, but NSAIDs are preferred if inflammation is present.
    - Doses should be administered on a scheduled basis, starting as early as possible in the course of the injury. A quick tapering of dose and dosing interval should occur as the injury improves (typically 1–3 days).
    - Adverse effects associated with oral NSAIDs include heartburn, dyspepsia, anorexia, epigastric pain, bleeding and bruising, and increased blood pressure.
    - Adverse effects associated with acetaminophen include nausea, hepato-toxicity, and skin rash (rare). It is well-tolerated when recommended doses are not exceeded.

CAUTIONS FOR NSAIDs

- Chronic use of NSAIDs can cause nephropathy, bleeding, increased cardiovascular events (e.g., MI, stroke, heart failure), and GI ulcerations, among other risks.
- GI risks are greatest in patients who are 60 years of age and older, have a history of peptic ulcer disease, consume 3 or more alcoholic beverages/day, and use higher doses, longer duration of treatment, or both.
- Risks may outweigh the benefits in patients 75 years and older; topical NSAIDs should be considered.

CAUTIONS FOR ACETAMINOPHEN

- Hepatoxicity can occur when doses exceed 4 g/day, particularly with chronic use.
- More conservative dosing (≤2 g/day) should be considered in the following patients: liver disease, concurrent hepatoxic drug(s), and 3 or more alcoholic beverages/day.
- Potential hidden sources of acetaminophen should be identified and discouraged (e.g., Tylenol PM).
- Manufacturer labeling has decreased the daily recommended dose for all patients to 3000–3250 mg/day to decrease the risk of accidental overdose.

Mild-moderate aches and pains (tendonitis, bursitis, sprains, strains) adjunct treatment of choice is topical analgesics.

- Topical Analgesics
  - Counterirritants
    - Topical counterirritants include camphor, capsaicin, menthol, methyl nicotinate, and methyl salicylate.
    - These are applied to the skin to relieve pain by producing a distracting, less severe pain.
    - Topical counterirritants should be applied to the affected area 3–4 times daily.
    - Pain relief with capsaicin use is delayed, with benefit emerging at 14 days and maximum relief sometimes taking 4–6 weeks. Use beyond 7 days with medical supervision is appropriate.

▫ Adverse effects associated with counterirritants include localized reactions (e.g., skin irritation, rash). Strong irritation can occur (e.g., erythema, blistering, thermal hyperalgesia, neurotoxicity).

CAUTIONS FOR COUNTERIRRITANTS

- These products have been associated with second- and third-degree burns.
- Products of greatest risk for burns are single-ingredient menthol or combination menthol (≥3%) and methyl salicylate (≥10%).
- Heat exposure (e.g., exercise directly after application) has been associated with a threefold increase in systemic absorption.
- Methyl salicylate should be used with caution in individuals with aspirin sensitivity.
- Menthol should be discontinued if the patient experiences rash, irritation, burning, stinging, swelling, or infection.
- Methyl nicotinate should not be applied over large areas of the body because of the risk of hypotension, bradycardia, and syncope.
- Capsaicin should not come in contact with the eyes or other mucus membranes.

- Topical Anesthetics
    ▫ Topical lidocaine cream and patches are available as nonprescription products.
    ▫ These are best used for nerve pain, which generally should not be treated without medical supervision.
    ▫ Patients should not exceed 3 applications in 24 hours.
    ▫ Adverse reactions associated with topical lidocaine include rash, itching, and skin irritation. If skin irritation occurs, the product should be removed and the area cleansed.

CAUTIONS FOR TOPICAL ANESTHETICS

- Systemic absorption can occur if applications exceed 3 times/day or are applied over broken skin.

- Trolamine Salicylate
    ▫ Trolamine salicylate does not have sufficient data to support its safety and efficacy in musculoskeletal conditions. Many commercially available products contain trolamine salicylate as a primary ingredient.

- Use of trolamine salicylate should be reserved for patients who do not tolerate or prefer the localized irritation of counterirritants.

CAUTIONS FOR TROLAMINE SALICYLATE

- Trolamine is absorbed through the skin and results in salicylate concentrations in the synovial. Excessive applications can pose the same risks as aspirin.

Osteoarthritis of hip and knee treatment of choice is acetaminophen.

- Acetaminophen
    - Acetaminophen is recommended as first-line therapy by the American College of Rheumatology (ACR).
    - Despite evidence that NSAIDs provide better pain relief, chronic daily use of NSAIDs leads to serious and prevalent adverse effects.
    - Adverse effects associated with acetaminophen include nausea, hepatotoxicity, and skin rash (rare). It is well-tolerated when recommended doses are not exceeded.

CAUTIONS FOR ACETAMINOPHEN

- Hepatoxicity can occur when doses exceed 4 g/day, particularly with chronic use.
- More conservative dosing (≤2 g/day) should be considered in the following patients: liver disease, concurrent hepatoxic drug(s), and 3 or more alcoholic beverages/day.
- Potential hidden sources of acetaminophen should be identified and discouraged (e.g., Tylenol PM).
- Manufacturer labeling has decreased the daily recommended dose for all patients to 3000–3250 mg/day to decrease the risk of accidental overdose.
- Rare but serious cutaneous adverse reactions have been associated with acetaminophen (Stevens-Johnson syndrome and toxic epidermal necrolysis). These reactions can be life-threatening. The medication should be stopped if any rash appears, and medical help should be sought right away.

- NSAIDs
    - NSAIDs are also appropriate treatment options for osteoarthritis according to ACR guidelines and can be considered.

- The American Association of Orthopedic Surgeons recommends oral or topical NSAIDs; however, the risks of NSAIDs must be considered.
- If used chronically, a proton pump inhibitor should be considered for GI protection.
- Adverse effects associated with oral NSAIDs include heartburn, dyspepsia, anorexia, epigastric pain, bleeding and bruising, and increased blood pressure.

CAUTIONS FOR NSAIDs

- Chronic use of NSAIDs can cause nephropathy, bleeding, increased cardiovascular events (e.g., MI, stroke, heart failure), and GI ulcerations, among other risks.
- GI risks are greatest in patients who are 60 years of age and older, have a history of peptic ulcer disease, consume 3 or more alcoholic beverages/day, and use higher doses, longer duration of treatment, or both.
- Risks may outweigh the benefits in patients 75 years and older; topical NSAIDs should be considered.

- Complementary Therapy
  - Glucosamine and chondroitin are the most commonly used supplements in osteoarthritis. Data are conflicting regarding joint space and pain relief. Current data suggest if a benefit will be derived, it is more likely in patients with moderate-severe pain. The ACR recommends that patients with osteoarthritis do not use these products.

Special Populations

No significant variability in response has been noted in patients of different ages.

- Pregnancy
  - Since complications can occur in pregnancy, patients should be evaluated by their health care provider or OB/GYN.
  - If the patient has been given approval by their health care provider for self-treatment, capsaicin and lidocaine are pregnancy Category B and can be considered.
    - It is suggested that topical camphor use is likely compatible with pregnancy.
  - Generally, NSAIDs should not be used in pregnancy unless it is clear that the potential benefit justifies the potential risk to the fetus.

NSAIDs are not known to be teratogenic but can cause prolonged labor and increased postpartum bleeding. They can also cause adverse fetal cardiovascular effects (e.g., premature closing of the ductus arteriosus). Risks of use are greatest in the third trimester.

- Acetaminophen crosses the placenta but is considered safe for pregnancy and is the first-line treatment for conditions that require oral systemic analgesics. Emerging evidence suggests there may be a slight association between maternal prenatal use of acetaminophen and attention deficit hyperactivity disorder (ADHD) in the child. Use for fewer than 8 days is negatively associated with ADHD. Use for more than 29 days has the greatest association. Patients should be advised of this potential association; however, short-term use appears nonsignificant.
- Aspirin can cross the placenta and poses both fetal and maternal harms. Thus, it should be avoided in pregnancy, particularly during the last semester.

- Breastfeeding
  - Capsaicin is thought to be transferred into breast milk.
  - Topical camphor is suggested as being compatible with breastfeeding, but data are limited.
  - Acetaminophen is considered compatible with breastfeeding but does appear in breast milk. The most common adverse effect in newborn exposure is a maculopapular rash that subsides upon discontinuation.
  - Naproxen should be avoided in nursing mothers. It is unknown if ibuprofen is excreted into breastmilk. Thus, ibuprofen use should be carefully weighed against potential harm to the infant.
  - Aspirin should be avoided during breastfeeding. No adverse effects via breast milk have been reported, but it is still considered to carry a risk.

- Pediatric Patients
  - Capsaicin should not be used in patients under 18 years of age.
  - External analgesics should not be used in children 2 years of age and older. Most products are labeled for 12 years of age and older.
    - Before using external agents in this patient population, it should be verified that the child can effectively communicate adverse effects.
    - Topical preparation of methyl salicylate should be avoided because of the risk of percutaneous absorption.
    - Topical camphor preparations are best avoided because of the risk of severe adverse reactions following accidental ingestion.

- Package labeling provides dosing of acetaminophen for children 2 years of age and older and ibuprofen for children 6 months of age and older, but pediatricians should be consulted first. Solid dosage forms do not provide dosing for use until 12 years of age.
- Salicylate-containing products (e.g., aspirin) should not be used in children under 12 years of age and adolescents, particularly those ill with influenza or chickenpox, because of the risk of Reye's Syndrome.

- Geriatric Patients
    - Before using external agents in older adult patients with memory or communication challenges, it should be verified that they do not impede their ability to effectively communicate adverse effects.

■ ■ QuES▣: Talk with the patient

● Patient Education/Counseling

- Nonpharmacologic Talking Points
    - RICE therapy is a cornerstone of musculoskeletal injury treatment and helps reduce swelling and inflammation:
        - <u>R</u>EST the injury and continue until pain is reduced (1–2 days).
        - <u>I</u>CE the injury as soon as possible for no more than 15–20–minute increments 3–4 times a day until swelling subsides (1–3 days).
            - Applying ice for more than 15–20 minutes causes vaso-constriction and can prolong the causative factors of the injury.
        - <u>C</u>OMPRESSION should be applied to the injury with elastic support or an elasticized bandage. The injury should be wrapped starting at the most distal point of the injury by overlapping the previous layer (1/3–1/2 previous width). Tightness of the bandage should be loosened as you wrap.
        - <u>E</u>LEVATE the injury at or above the heart level to decrease swelling and relieve pain.
    - Heat therapy may be used for noninflammatory injuries to relieve stiffness. Heat should be applied for 15–20 minutes, 3–4 times a day.
        - This should not be used with topical analgesics, areas with decreased sensation, over broken skin, or on inflamed areas.
        - Heat should not be applied to inflamed areas because it can worsen injury.
        - Heating devices should not be applied to skin with decreased sensation or during sleep because of the risk of burns.

  - Heat can be applied as warm wet compresses, a heating pad, a hot water bottle, or heat-generation adhesive and wrap products (e.g., ThermaCare).
- Transcutaneous electrical nerve stimulation (TENS) units are now available without a prescription and can be used for 15–30 minutes up to 3 times daily. Electrodes should not be placed on open wounds, rashes, inflamed skin, cancerous lesions, skin with altered sensation, areas treated with topical analgesics, throat, chest, head, or over the carotid arteries.
  - Pregnant patients, patients with internal or attached medical devices (e.g., pacemakers), and pediatric patients should not use nonprescription TENS units.

- Pharmacologic Talking Points
  - Systemic Analgesics
    - Patients should be reminded of the maximum dosages of nonprescription analgesic treatment:
      - Ibuprofen maximum dose is 1200 mg/day.
      - Naproxen sodium maximum dose is 660 mg/day.
      - Acetaminophen maximum dose is 3000–3250 mg/day.
    - Oral analgesics are scheduled for greatest pain relief.
  - Topical Analgesics
    - Patients should wash their hands before and after applying all topical preparations to avoid adverse effects on mucosal membranes, particularly capsaicin.
    - Topical preparations should not be applied to skin that is broken or damaged.
    - Topical preparations should be used carefully with adjunct therapies, such as heat and wrapping. These should be separated by several hours to avoid burns and systemic absorption.
    - Topical counterirritants produce a mild local inflammation that causes localized redness and warmth or coolness. This provides symptomatic relief to mask the pain at the site.
      - Medical attention should be sought if burning or blistering occurs.
    - Patients with young children in the house should ensure these are stored in a nonvisible, nonaccessible area, as these can be toxic when ingested.

- Suggest medical referral if any of the following occur:
  - Pain does not show improvement after 7 days of treatment with topical analgesics

- Pain does not show improvement after 10 days of treatment with oral analgesics
- Pain lasts over 10 days regardless of treatment
- Burns or significant topical irritation are suspected

Clinical Pearls

- Topical analgesics are used as an adjunct or substitute to oral pharmaco-therapy.

- Cost, ease of use, dosage form, and odor of the preparation should be considered and discussed with the patient before selecting a therapy.

- In general, the lowest effective dose should be recommended for the shortest duration needed.

- Postexercise icing is often appropriate to reduce the likelihood of inflammation and reduce pain.

- While the reason is unclear, some patients will report a better response to one NSAID than another. Thus, if a patient fails one NSAID, a trial with another nonprescription NSAID can be recommended.

- It is irrational to combine topical counterirritants with local anesthetics or local analgesics. Local anesthetics or analgesics can depress sensory cutaneous reports, opposing the counterirritant stimulation of these receptors.

References

1. Olenak JL. Musculoskeletal injuries and disorders. In: Krinsky DL, Ferreri SP, Hemstreet BA, Hume AL, Newton GD, Rollins CJ, Tietze KJ, eds. *Handbook of Nonprescription Drugs: An Interactive Approach to Self-Care*. Washington, DC: American Pharmacists Association; 2017:111–130.

Additional References

1. Wilkinson JJ, Tromp K. Headache. In: Krinsky DL, Ferreri SP, Hemstreet BA, Hume AL, Newton GD, Rollins CJ, Tietze KJ, eds. *Handbook of Nonprescription Drugs: An Interactive Approach to Self-Care*. Washington, DC: American Pharmacists Association; 2017:77–110.

2. Ystrom E, Gustavson K, Brandlistuen RE, et al. Prenatal exposure to acetaminophen and risk of ADHD. *Pediatrics*. 2017;140(5):e20163840.

PEDICULOSIS

Rashi Chandra Waghel, PharmD, BCACP
and Jennifer A. Wilson, PharmD, BCACP

For complete information about this topic, consult Chapter 37, "Insect Bites and Stings and Pediculosis," written by Patricia H. Fabel and Elizabeth Weeks Blake and published in the *Handbook of Nonprescription Drugs*, 19th Edition.[1]

Self-Care of Pediculosis

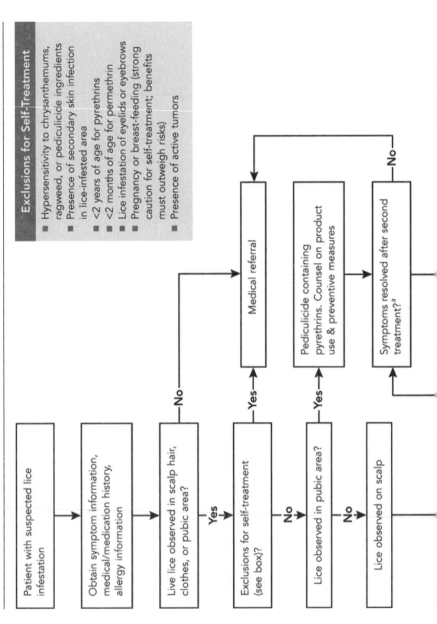

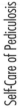

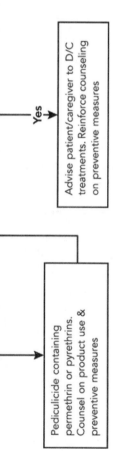

Yes

Advise patient/caregiver to D/C treatments. Reinforce counseling on preventive measures

Pediculicide containing permethrin or pyrethrins. Counsel on product use & preventive measures

ª Permethrin rinse has residual effects for up to 10 days. Retreatment in 7–10 days is not required unless active lice are detected. D/C = discontinue.

■■ Overview

■ Lice infestations commonly occur in the United States. There are three types of lice infestations, most commonly including head (*Pediculus humanus capitis*) as well as body (*Pediculus humanus corporis*) and pubic (*Phthirus pubis*).

■ Outbreaks most commonly occur in schools and daycares during the fall months and can affect all socioeconomic classes.

■ The goal of self-treatment is to eradicate the infestation (both lice and nits) and limit transmission.

■■ Pathophysiology

■ Adult lice lay eggs ("nits"), which hatch and must begin feeding within 24 hours. It takes 8–9 days for newly hatched lice to mature. If left untreated, the cycle repeats every 3 weeks.

■ Transmission

■ Head lice are generally spread by close personal contact with infected persons or sharing of personal items (e.g., combs, brushes, towels, hats) and are not a result of poor hygiene.

■ Poor hygiene (e.g., not showering or changing clothes on a frequent basis) can contribute to the transmission of body lice.

■ Pubic lice (i.e., "crabs") are usually spread through sexual contact with an infected person or sharing of personal items. It should be noted that while these infestations often occur in the pubic region, they may also affect other areas (e.g., armpits, eyelashes, facial hair).

■ Preventative Measures

■ Avoiding direct contact with infected individuals and their personal items can help to prevent further transmission and spread.

■■ QuEST: Quickly and Accurate Assess the Patient Using SCHOLAR MAC

QuEST SCHOLAR is an acronym used to assess a patient to determine self-care candidate status and to identify which treatment would be most appropriate. See Chapter 1 for a description of the QuEST SCHOLAR process.

Does the Patient Have Pediculosis?

- A papule will develop within 24 hours of being bitten by a louse.

- Itching is the predominant symptom, which can lead to scratching. Scratching can potentially result in a secondary bacterial infection.

Important SCHOLAR MAC Considerations

- Where on the body is the lice infestation?
    - Location is important in determining if a patient is a candidate for self-care and, if so, for choosing an appropriate pediculicide treatment option.

- What previous lice therapies have been used and how recently?
    - Previous treatment and time since last treatment will determine if the patient is a candidate for self-care and will guide selection of appropriate pediculicide treatment.

Physical Assessment Techniques

- For suspected head lice infestations, inspect the crown of the head, around the ears, and the base of the neck for live lice, nits, and nit casings. Nits are grayish and can often blend with hair, whereas nit casings are lighter in color. Firm attachment to the hair shaft will help differentiate nit casings from dandruff or dirt. Adult lice can be more difficult to detect because of movement, but lice feces may be visible (black, powdery specks).

- Visually inspect for local papules, which are often found near the site of bites.

- For suspected body lice infestations, inspect the seams and folds of clothing for live lice, nits, and nit casings.

- For suspected pubic lice infestations, patient should be instructed to inspect the pubic region, as well as armpits, eyelashes, and facial hair for presence of live lice, nits, and nit casings.

- **It is important that the presence of lice be confirmed by observation prior to initiating any treatment to help reduce emerging resistance to available products.**

◼ ◼ QuⒺST: Establish that the patient is an appropriate self-care candidate

Utilize the information collected in the patient assessment with the treatment algorithm and exclusions for self-care to determine if self-care is appropriate.

◼ Exclusions for Self-Care

Review the treatment algorithm and exclusions for self-care provided at the beginning of the chapter. This section highlights key exclusion criteria.

◼ Medications

- ▪ Concurrent medications do not factor into treatment decisions.

◼ Allergies

- ▪ Individuals with a hypersensitivity to chrysanthemums should avoid use of synergized pyrethrins (derived from chrysanthemum flowers) and permethrin, a synthetic pyrethroid.

- ▪ Ragweed-sensitive individuals should avoid synergized pyrethrins, as they may experience cross-sensitivity, as they are related plants.

◼ Conditions

- ▪ Individuals who exhibit signs or symptoms of secondary bacterial skin infections in the area of the infestation (e.g., erythema, swelling, presence of pus, broken skin) should be referred to their primary care provider to address the infection.

◼ Special Populations

- ▪ Women who are pregnant or breastfeeding should avoid self-treatment of pediculosis.

◼ ◼ QuE**S**T: Suggest appropriate self-care strategies

Select the appropriate treatment option based on the previously collected patient data. Various treatment options are discussed along with clinical pearls and pertinent patient considerations for optimal management.

◼ Treatment Options

Lice treatment of choice is a pediculicide.

- ▪ Pediculicides
    - ▫ These agents will eradicate nits and live lice.
    - ▫ The two ingredients approved for self-care use as a pediculicide are synergized pyrethrins and permethrin.

- Synergized pyrethrins are approved for treatment of head and pubic lice to improve efficacy.
- Permethrin 1% is available as a topical cream rinse and is approved for self-treatment of head lice only.
- Adverse effects associated with both synergized pyrethrins and permethrin include local irritation (e.g., burning, stinging, itching), erythema, and swelling.

CAUTIONS FOR PEDICULICIDES

- Avoid oral ingestion and contact with eyes and other mucous membranes.
- Avoid exceeding recommended application times or occluding the treated area while product is applied, as this may increase absorption and therefore increase risk of adverse effects.

Other Treatment Considerations

- There are emerging therapies for those looking for pesticide-free products as well as those who are in regions that have high resistance to nonprescription pediculicides.
- The Nuvo method, using Cetaphil cleanser, is a dry-on, suffocation-based pediculicide. The cleanser is applied to the hair and dried to suffocate and eradicate the lice.
- Dimethicone 100% gel is another pesticide-free option that coats the lice and immobilizes them. It may cause less irritation than traditional pediculicides.
- AirAllé (formerly called the LouseBuster) is a machine that uses heat to dehydrate lice and nits. However, its use may be cost prohibitive, and it requires a certified technician for operation.
- Battery-operated louse combs, which claim to kill lice, are also available. However, there is no evidence to support use at this time, and these products should not be used in patients with pacemakers or seizures.

Complementary Therapy

- Lice enzyme shampoos are another alternative treatment option. They are thought to break down the lice exoskeleton, resulting in eradication of the infestation. One studied product contains 10% tree oil and 1% lavender oil, which is applied weekly for three weeks. It should be noted that tea tree oil can potentially cause significant allergic reactions or liver toxicity.

- *Natrum muriaticum* (sodium chloride), when applied to dry hair for 15 minutes, dries out lice and eggs.
- Other oil-based products (e.g., petroleum jelly, mayonnaise) have not been proven to be very effective in eradicating lice by suffocation.

Special Populations

- Pediatric Patients
    - Products containing synergized pyrethrins should not be used on children less than 2 years of age. Products containing permethrins should not be used on infants less than 2 months of age.
    - Skin protectants can be used on children less than 2 years of age.

QuES T: Talk with the patient

Patient Education/Counseling

- Nonpharmacologic Talking Points
    - Nonpharmacologic measures are important in the treatment of lice infestation to help prevent reoccurrence and reduce spread.
    - It is important to visually inspect the hair for remaining nits and utilize a nit comb, since the pediculicide products do not kill 100% of all lice eggs.
    - Direct contact with an infected individual or any infected objects (e.g., combs, towels, hats) should be avoided.
    - Though labor intensive, it is important to eliminate lice and nits from any infected objects to avoid reinfestation. These measures should be in addition to proper pharmacologic treatment.
    - Washable items, such as toys, brushes, and combs, should be soaked in hot water (≥130°F) for 10 minutes. Bedding, towels, and clothes should be washed in hot water (≥130°F) and dried using the hottest setting recommended for the fabric.
    - Items that cannot be washed should be sealed in plastic bag for at least 2 weeks.
    - Furniture and carpet should be thoroughly vacuumed regularly throughout the treatment period; insecticidal sprays are not generally recommended.
- Pharmacologic Talking Points
    - Synergized Pyrethrins
        - Apply product to dry hair. Let it sit on the hair for 10 minutes, then work into a lather and rinse thoroughly.

- Use a nit comb after treatment to remove dead lice and nits.
- A second application is required 7–10 days later to eradicate any remaining nits that have hatched.
  - Permethrin
    - Apply product to wet, freshly shampooed hair that has been towel dried. Let it sit on the hair for 10 minutes; rinse thoroughly and dry hair.
    - Use a nit comb to remove dead lice and nits.
    - A second application of permethrin is only required if active lice are observed 7–10 days later.

- Suggest medical referral if any of the following occur:
  - If signs of infestation still exist after the second application of the pediculicide, medical referral is recommended.
  - In regions with high resistance to nonprescription pediculicides, referral to a healthcare provider for a prescription pediculicide may be more appropriate.

Clinical Pearls

- Follow up should occur within 10 days. Patients should seek medical attention if signs of infestation still persist after a second application of pediculicide.

- Since resistance rates against pediculicide products are increasing, overuse of products should be avoided. Visual inspection confirming the presence of lice or nits is important before applying any pediculicide product.

- Nonpharmacologic measures should be emphasized to help avoid reinfestation or spread of lice.

- Alternative therapies or medical referral could be considered for patients in regions of high resistance to nonprescription pediculicides.

References

1. Fabel PH and Blake EW. Insect bites and stings and pediculosis. In: Krinsky DL, Ferreri SP, Henstreet BA, Hume AL, Newton GD, Rollins CJ, Tietze KJ, eds. *Handbook of Nonprescription Drugs: An Interactive Approach to Self-Care*. Washington, DC: American Pharmacists Association; 2017:709–725.

SCALY DERMATOSES

Cortney M. Mospan, PharmD, BCACP, BCGP

For complete information about this topic, consult Chapter 34, "Scaly Dermatoses," written by Rupal Patel Mansukhani and Lucio Volino and published in the *Handbook of Nonprescription Drugs*, 19th Edition.[1]

Self-Care of Scaly Dermatoses

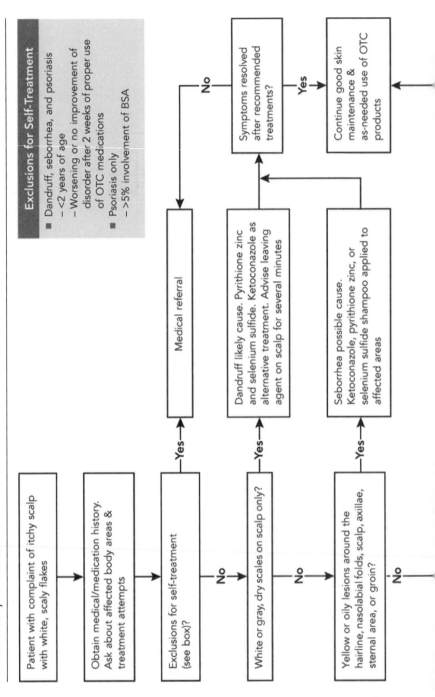

Exclusions for Self-Treatment

- Dandruff, seborrhea, and psoriasis
  - <2 years of age
  - Worsening or no improvement of disorder after 2 weeks of proper use of OTC medications
- Psoriasis only
  - >5% involvement of BSA

Patient with complaint of itchy scalp with white, scaly flakes

Obtain medical/medication history. Ask about affected body areas & treatment attempts

Exclusions for self-treatment (see box)? — Yes → Medical referral — No → Symptoms resolved after recommended treatments? — Yes → Continue good skin maintenance & as-needed use of OTC products

White or gray, dry scales on scalp only? — Yes → Dandruff likely cause. Pyrithione zinc and selenium sulfide. Ketoconazole as alternative treatment. Advise leaving agent on scalp for several minutes — No →

Yellow or oily lesions around the hairline, nasolabial folds, scalp, axillae, sternal area, or groin? — Yes → Seborrhea possible cause. Ketoconazole, pyrithione zinc, or selenium sulfide shampoo applied to affected areas — No →

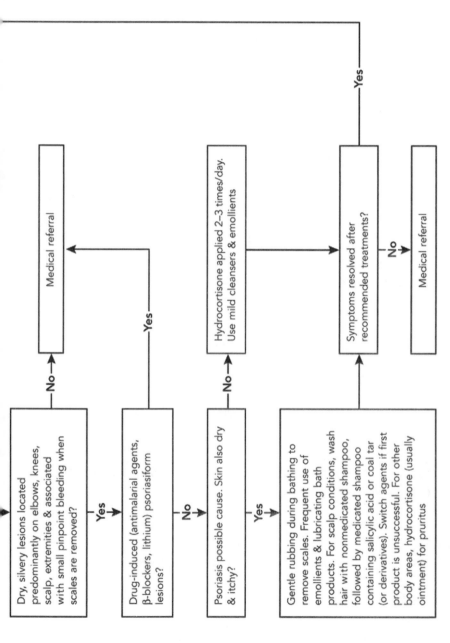

BSA = body surface area; OTC = over-the-counter.

■ ■ Overview

- Scaly dermatoses is a chronic condition that includes dandruff, seborrheic dermatitis, and psoriasis.

- Nonprescription products are appropriate treatments in most cases of dandruff and seborrheic dermatitis. While mild psoriasis may be responsive to nonprescription products, initial diagnosis and acute flares require primary care provider or dermatologist attention.

- Goals of treatment include decreasing epidermal cell turnover rate, minimizing cosmetic embarrassment, relief of any itching, and prevention of flare-ups.

■ ■ Pathophysiology

- Dandruff is a hyperproliferative condition with accelerated epidermal cell turnover and abnormal keratinization that produces inflammation, flaking, and itching. This process results from the presence of *Malassezia* yeast.

- Seborrheic dermatitis also involves *Malassezia* yeast with accelerated epidermal proliferation. Generally, areas with dense concentration of sebaceous glands exhibit greater inflammation.

- Psoriasis can be triggered by environmental factors, infections, prescription drug use, stress, obesity, and alcohol and tobacco use. Psoriasis lesions are often localized but can become generalized over large portions of the body.
  - Remissions and exacerbations are unpredictable and can result in significant psychological and physical distress. Immunologic functions are thought to contribute to the development and exacerbation of psoriasis.

■ ■ QuEST: Quickly and Accurate Assess the Patient Using SCHOLAR MAC

QuEST SCHOLAR is an acronym used to assess a patient to determine self-care candidate status and to identify which treatment would be most appropriate. See Chapter 1 for a description of the QuEST SCHOLAR process.

■ Does the Patient Have Dandruff?

- Scalp scaling and sloughing off of small white or gray loose flakes is the only visible manifestation of dandruff.

■ Additional but less common symptoms include scalp itching, dryness, irritation, and tightness. Generally, no visible inflammation or erythema will be present.

Does the Patient Have Seborrheic Dermatitis?

■ Seborrheic dermatitis occurs predominantly in the areas of greatest sebaceous gland activity (e.g., chest, scalp, face). It can affect the scalp, eyebrows and between the eyebrows, eyelid margins, cheeks, paranasal areas, nasolabial folds, beard area, parasternal area, central back, creases behind the ear, and ear canal.

■ Commonly presents as a red, itchy, scaly rash. The most common presentation is yellow, well-demarcated, greasy, oily scales on the scalp or plaques, exudation, and thick crusting.
  ▪ In children, this is commonly referred to as "cradle cap," with thick white to yellow-brown greasy scales on the scalp that can extend to the face, neck, trunk, and extremities.
  ▪ In adults, it is a chronic condition that is typically more severe in the winter, low-humidity environments, and times of stress. Yellow, greasy scales are present on the scalp that can extend to the face with eyebrow involvement.

Does the Patient Have Psoriasis?

■ Psoriasis lesions start as small papules that grow into raised plaques, which typically have thick silvery white scales. Plaques may be painful or itchy.

■ Psoriasis typically presents symmetrically. Common locations include the extensor surfaces of knees and elbows, lumbar region of the back, scalp, trunk, and genital area.

■ Table 1 provides a comparison of key symptom differences between dandruff, seborrheic dermatitis, and psoriasis.

Important SCHOLAR MAC Considerations

■ Where are the symptoms located (e.g., head, chest, elbows)?
  ▪ Appropriate treatment will vary based on which type of scaly dermatoses the patient has. Locations of the symptoms can help determine the type of scaly dermatoses and subsequent treatment.

TABLE 1. Distinguishing features of scaly dermatoses

	Dandruff	Seborrheic Dermatitis	Psoriasis
Location	Scalp	Scalp, face, trunk	Scalp, elbows, knees, trunk, lower extremities
Exacerbating factors	Generally a stable condition, but may be exacerbated by psychological stress, cold temperatures, dry climate	Immunosuppression, neurologic conditions, environment, stress	Environmental factors, infection, medications, stress, obesity, alcohol, tobacco
Appearance	Thin, white, or grayish flakes; even distribution on scalp	Macules, patches, and thin plaques of discrete yellow oily scales on red skin	Discrete symmetrical red plaques with sharp borders; silvery white scales; small bleeding points when scales are removed; difficult to distinguish from seborrhea in early stages or in intertriginous zones
Inflammation	Absent	Present	Present
Epidermal hyperplasia	Absent	Present	Present
Epidermal kinetics	Turnover rate 2 times faster than normal	Turnover rate about 3 times faster than normal	Turnover rate about 8 times faster than normal

- Is inflammation or erythema present?
  - Dandruff generally does not have visible inflammation or erythema, which helps to identify scaly dermatoses type and subsequent treatment.
  - Severe inflammation and erythema likely will not be resolved with nonprescription medications.

■ ■ Qu❶ST: Establish that the patient is an appropriate self-care candidate

Utilize the information collected in the patient assessment with the treatment algorithm and exclusions for self-care to determine if self-care is appropriate.

■ Exclusions to Self-Care

Review the treatment algorithm and exclusions for self-care provided at the beginning of the chapter. This section highlights key exclusion criteria.

■ Medications

- Psoriasis can be exacerbated by medication use—patients using the following medications should be referred to their primary care provider or dermatologist: antimalarials, beta blockers, interferons, lithium, and nonsteroidal anti-inflammatory drugs (NSAIDs), as well as patients experiencing systemic corticosteroid withdrawal.

◼ Conditions

◼ Psoriasis covering 5% or more of the patient's body surface area requires referral, as systemic adverse effects can occur with nonprescription products applied over a large surface area.

◼ Special Populations

◼ Children less than 2 years of age should be referred because of higher absorption of topical therapies.

◼ ◼ QuE⑤T: Suggest appropriate self-care strategies

Select the appropriate treatment option based on the previously collected patient data. Various treatment options are discussed along with clinical pearls and pertinent patient considerations for optimal management.

◼ Treatment Options

Dandruff treatment of choice is medicated shampoo with a cytostatic agent.

◼ Cytostatic Medicated Shampoos
- ◾ Cytostatic agents (e.g., pyrithione zinc, selenium sulfide) are the recommended initial treatment selection.
- ◾ Patients can follow treatment with use of a nonmedicated shampoo to reduce odor of the treatment shampoo.
- ◾ Pyrithione zinc and selenium sulfide are generally well tolerated without any significant adverse effects.

> **CAUTIONS FOR CYTOSTATIC MEDICATED SHAMPOOS**
> - ◾ Repeated rinsing (2–3 times) is recommended with selenium sulfide products to avoid leftover residue that can cause discoloration.
> - ◾ Contact with the eyes should be avoided to prevent stinging.

◼ Antifungal Medicated Shampoos
- ◾ Nonprescription antifungal shampoos include ketoconazole.
- ◾ This can be an alternative treatment selection to a cytostatic agent.

- Adverse effects of ketoconazole shampoo include skin irritation, hair loss, abnormal hair texture, and dry skin.

> ### CAUTIONS FOR ANTIFUNGAL MEDICATED SHAMPOOS
> - Contact with the eyes should be avoided to prevent stinging.

- General-Purpose Nonmedicated Shampoo
  - Daily to every other day use of a routine shampoo product is sufficient for mild-moderate dandruff.

> ### CAUTIONS FOR NONMEDICATED SHAMPOOS
> - Shampoos with harsh surfactants (e.g., sodium lauryl sulfate, sodium laureth sulfate) should be avoided because of damaging effects to skin layers.

- Keratolytic Medicated Shampoo
  - Nonprescription keratolytic shampoos include salicylic acid and sulfur.
  - These should be a second-line recommendation if patients dislike or cannot tolerate other shampoos, as they have limited benefit and require longer treatment duration.

> ### CAUTIONS FOR KERATOLYTIC SHAMPOOS
> - Application over extensive areas should be avoided because of the potential for percutaneous absorption of salicylic acid.

- Coal Tar Shampoos
  - Shampoos with coal tar are generally reserved as a final second-line therapy because of discoloration of hair, skin and scalp, and clothing.
  - Adverse effects of coal tar include folliculitis, stains to skin and hair, irritant contact dermatitis, and photosensitization.

> ### CAUTIONS FOR COAL TAR SHAMPOOS
> - Photosensitization can occur. Patients using coal tar preparations should avoid sun exposure for 24 hours after application.

Adult seborrheic dermatitis lesion treatment of choice is medicated shampoo.

■ Medicated Shampoos
- Shampooing is the foundation of treatment in adults, regardless of the location of the skin lesion.
- Topical antifungals (ketoconazole) are first-line for treatment of seborrheic dermatitis.
- Since seborrheic dermatitis is a chronic condition, other cytostatic agents (pyrithione zinc and selenium sulfide) can be used as well.
- If the odor of a mediated shampoo is undesirable, it can be followed by a more cosmetically acceptable shampoo or conditioner.
- Nonmedicated shampoos can be used to soften and remove crusts or scales.
- Adverse effects of ketoconazole shampoo include skin irritation, hair loss, abnormal hair texture, and dry skin. Pyrithione zinc and selenium sulfide are generally well-tolerated.

Adult seborrheic dermatitis inflammation and itching treatment of choice is topical corticosteroid ointment.

■ Topical Corticosteroid
- Hydrocortisone can be used when erythema persists after medicated shampoo use.
- While not useful in treating dandruff, topical corticosteroids are needed in seborrheic dermatitis to treat the greater level of inflammation.
- Adverse effects associated with topical corticosteroids include burning and atrophy.

> **CAUTIONS FOR TOPICAL CORTICOSTEROIDS**
> - Systemic absorption is minimal when used on intact skin but can occur when applied over large surface areas, with prolonged use, with occlusive dressing, or when skin integrity is compromised.
> - Local tissue atrophy can occur with prolonged use.
> - Aggravation can occur when used on cutaneous infections.

Psoriasis treatment of choice for dry skin is topical emollients.

■ Topical Emollients
- Products included as emollients include lotions and creams (e.g., Lubriderm Lotion and Nivea Creme) as well as lubricating bath products.

- Daily lubrication of the skin after a bath or shower is essential and should be applied within minutes of showering or bathing.
- To be effective, these products need to be applied up to 4 times daily. However, these measures alone are unlikely to control signs and symptoms of psoriasis.

Psoriasis treatment of choice for red and inflamed lesions is topical corticosteroids.

- ■ Topical Corticosteroid
    - Hydrocortisone 1% ointment is the drug of choice in patients with bright red lesions, but some patients may require more potent prescription corticosteroids.
    - Efficacy can be enhanced by covering the area 30 minutes after hydrocortisone application via occlusion with a greasy emollient (e.g., petrolatum).
    - Adverse effects associated with topical corticosteroids include burning and atrophy.

● Special Populations

- ■ Pediatric Patients
    - Cradle cap is the infantile form of seborrheic dermatitis that occurs in the first 3 months of life. This condition is usually self-limited.
    - This can be treated by gently massaging the scalp with baby oil, followed by a nonmedicated shampoo (e.g., Johnson's baby shampoo, Mustela Foam shampoo) to loosen scales.

■ ● QuEST: Talk with the patient

● Patient Education/Counseling

- ■ Nonpharmacologic Talking Points
    - Patients should be educated that treatment of scaly dermatoses focuses on controlling the condition, not curing it. Thus, selected therapies need to be ongoing for adequate control.
    - Patients with psoriasis should avoid physical, chemical, or ultraviolet (UV) skin trauma because of a high likelihood of developing lesions at the site.
    - Patients with psoriasis should bathe with lubricating bath products 2–3 times per week with tepid water.

- Patients should be made aware that seborrheic dermatitis and psoriasis generally fluctuate as a result of emotional, physical, and environmental factors. Plans should be developed to minimize exposure to triggers and strategies provided to help minimize exacerbations.

- Pharmacologic Talking Points
  - Medicated Shampoos
    - Patients should shampoo with nonmedicated, nonresidue shampoo to remove dirt, oil, and scales from scalp and hair before use of a medicated shampoo. Nonmedicated shampoos can leave a residue on the hair shaft that can aggravate the condition.
    - The shampoo should be massaged onto the scalp (affected area and surrounding) with a scalp scrubber, if possible, and left on the hair for 3–5 minutes. Contact time is essential for these products to slow replication of the *Malassezia* species. Scalp scrubbers are useful, particularly in patients with longer hair, to ensure adequate contact with the scalp.
    - Shampoos should be used daily for 1 week, then 2–3 times weekly, then once weekly or every other week for dandruff.
    - Shampoos should be used daily for 1–2 weeks, then 2–3 times weekly for 4 weeks for seborrheic dermatitis. Once the condition is controlled, the shampoo should be applied once weekly to prevent relapse.
      - If possible, should taper to the lowest effective dose
  - Topical Corticosteroids
    - Hydrocortisone ointment should be applied as a thin layer no more than twice daily and for no more than 7 consecutive days. Prolonged (>7 days) use can cause rebound flare-ups when discontinued.
  - Topical Emollients
    - Emollients should be applied liberally with gentle rubbing up to 4 times daily. Loose scales can be removed with a soft cloth.

- Suggest medical referral if any of the following occur:
  - Patients whose dandruff is resistant to nonprescription medicated shampoos should be referred to a primary care provider for further evaluation.
  - Infants that do not respond to nonmedicated shampoo treatment of cradle cap should be referred to their pediatrician.

- Condition does not improve or worsens after two weeks of treatment with nonprescription medications
  - If the condition worsens or symptoms persist longer than 7 days, a primary care provider or dermatologist should be consulted, as a more potent prescription corticosteroid may be indicated.
  - Follow-up should occur 1 week after self-treatment. If the condition has not worsened and is improving, the patient should return at 2 weeks. If symptoms persist or worsen, the patient should be referred to a primary care provider.
- Patients with psoriasis who have more than 5% body surface area affected, involvement of the face, or joint pain should be referred for more effective therapies.

Clinical Pearls

- Selection of product should be based on consideration of the patient's history, previous therapies used, and responses to those therapies.

References

1. Mansukhani RP, Volino L. Scaly dermatoses. In: Krinsky DL, Ferreri SP, Hemstreet BA, Hume AL, Newton GD, Rollins CJ, Tietze KJ, eds. *Handbook of Nonprescription Drugs: An Interactive Approach to Self-Care*. Washington, DC: American Pharmacists Association; 2017:667–679.

Additional References

1. Darbshire PL, Plake KS. Contact dermatitis. In: Krinsky DL, Ferreri SP, Hemstreet BA, Hume AL, Newton GD, Rollins CJ, Tietze KJ, eds. *Handbook of Nonprescription Drugs: An Interactive Approach to Self-Care*. Washington, DC: American Pharmacists Association; 2017:681–694.

TOBACCO CESSATION

Cortney M. Mospan, PharmD, BCACP, BCGP

For complete information about this topic, consult Chapter 47, "Tobacco Cessation," written by Beth A. Martin and Marcia C. Wopat and published in the *Handbook of Nonprescription Drugs*, 19th Edition.[1]

Self-Care of Tobacco Cessation

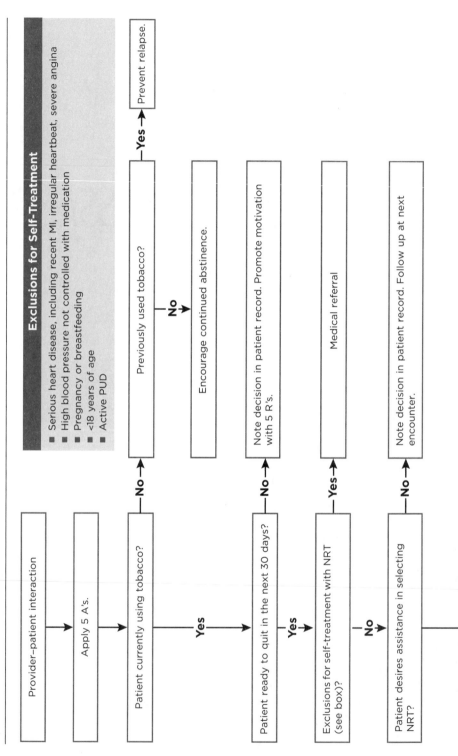

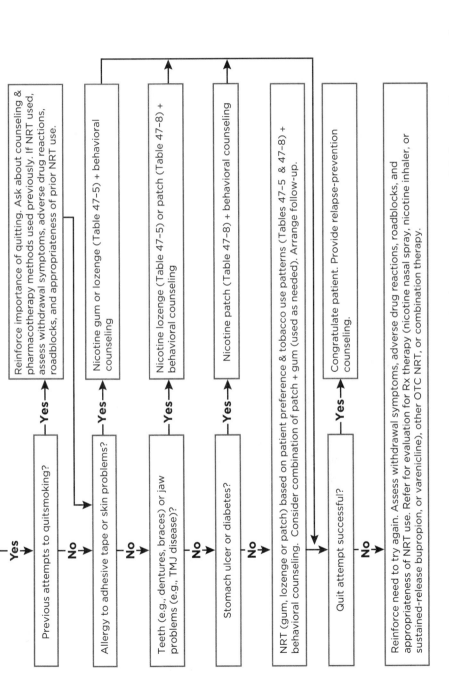

Yes

Previous attempts to quit smoking? —**Yes**→ Reinforce importance of quitting. Ask about counseling & pharmacotherapy methods used previously. If NRT used, assess withdrawal symptoms, adverse drug reactions, roadblocks, and appropriateness of prior NRT use.

No

Allergy to adhesive tape or skin problems? —**Yes**→ Nicotine gum or lozenge (Table 47-5) + behavioral counseling

No

Teeth (e.g., dentures, braces) or jaw problems (e.g. TMJ disease)? —**Yes**→ Nicotine lozenge (Table 47-5) or patch (Table 47-8) + behavioral counseling

No

Stomach ulcer or diabetes? —**Yes**→ Nicotine patch (Table 47-8) + behavioral counseling

No

NRT (gum, lozenge or patch) based on patient preference & tobacco use patterns (Tables 47-5 & 47-8) + behavioral counseling. Consider combination of patch + gum (used as needed). Arrange follow-up.

Quit attempt successful? —**Yes**→ Congratulate patient. Provide relapse-prevention counseling.

No

Reinforce need to try again. Assess withdrawal symptoms, adverse drug reactions, roadblocks, and appropriateness of NRT use. Refer for evaluation for Rx therapy (nicotine nasal spray, nicotine inhaler, or sustained-release bupropion, or varenicline), other OTC NRT, or combination therapy.

5 A's = Ask, advise, assess, assist, arrange; 5 R's = relevance, risks, rewards, roadblocks, repetition. MI = myocardial infarction; NRT = nicotine replacement therapy; OTC = over-the-counter; PUD = peptic ulcer disease; Rx = prescription; TMJ = temporomandibular joint.

■ ■ Overview

- Tobacco use is the leading cause of preventable death, responsible for nearly 480,000 deaths a year.

- Most patients who smoke quit cold turkey, with 95% of attempts ending in relapse. Patients who receive assistance in quitting have increased odds of quitting.
    - Patients are 1.7 times as likely to quit and remain tobacco free at over 5 months with intervention from nonphysician health care providers, such as pharmacists.
    - Even minimal interventions (<3 minutes) increase cessation rates.

- The primary goal of tobacco cessation treatment is long-term abstinence from all nicotine-containing products.

■ ■ Pathophysiology

- Tobacco dependence has similar underlying pharmacologic and behavioral processes as addiction to drugs like heroin and cocaine.

- Nicotine stimulates the mesolimbic dopaminergic system or the dopamine reward pathway, inducing pleasant or rewarding effects that promote continued use.

- Nicotine activates nicotinic cholinergic receptors, causing release of numerous neurotransmitters, resulting in pleasure, appetite suppression, cognitive enhancement, arousal, mood modulation, learning and memory enhancement, and anxiety and tension reduction.

- Psychosocial, behavioral, genetic, and environmental factors have a role in tobacco dependence. Smoking is commonly associated with specific activities (e.g., driving, drinking coffee, being around others who smoke), resulting in routines that can be difficult to break.

■ Clinical Presentation of Tobacco Use and Dependence

- Most chronic tobacco users will develop tolerance to the effects of nicotine, with abrupt cessation resulting in withdrawal symptoms.

- Withdrawal symptoms present within 1–2 days, peak within a week, and typically dissipate by 2–4 weeks.

- Symptoms and severity vary but can include irritability, frustration, anger, anxiety, depression, difficulty concentrating, impatience, insomnia, restlessness, and cravings. Increased appetite and weight gain may persist for 6 months after quitting or beyond.

■ ■ ◖Qu◗EST: Quickly and Accurate Assess the Patient Using SCHOLAR MAC

QuEST SCHOLAR is an acronym used to assess a patient to determine self-care candidate status and to identify which treatment would be most appropriate. See Chapter 1 for a description of the QuEST SCHOLAR process.

● *Does the Patient Qualify for Nonprescription Smoking Cessation Therapy?*

- It is not appropriate to recommend a treatment regimen until a patient is ready to quit (within the next month).

- If patients are ready to quit, therapy should be recommended with a quit date.

- The following should be discussed:
    - Cigarettes/day
    - Previous quit methods

● *Important SCHOLAR MAC Considerations*

- Have there been previous quit attempts?
    - What counseling and pharmacotherapy methods were used? Were they effective? Were there issues?
    - What withdrawal symptoms, adverse drug reactions, and roadblocks occurred?
    - A quit plan should be developed that addresses previous challenges and avoids ineffective therapies.

- How many cigarettes does the patient smoke a day?
    - Pharmacotherapy is recommended by treatment guidelines in patients who smoke 10 or more cigarettes a day. Behavioral interventions only should be used for patients who smoke less than 10 cigarettes a day.
    - Nicotine patches are approved for use in light smokers.
    - Nicotine lozenges have been found to be effective in patients who smoke 15 or fewer cigarettes a day.
    - Use of nicotine replacement therapy (NRT) in patients who smoke less than 10 cigarettes should be weighed for benefit in individual patients as a motivator.

Physical and Behavioral Assessment Techniques

- Observe the patient for signs of chronic medical conditions, such as wheezing (chronic obstructive pulmonary disease [COPD]), productive cough (COPD), and barrel chest (COPD).

- Obtain vital signs (e.g., pulse, blood pressure) to verify NRT is safe for self-care treatment.

- The 5 A's Approach
  - This comprehensive counseling approach should be the foundation of assessing patients' readiness to quit smoking.
  - Wording is key so that occasional smokers and nontraditional nicotine and tobacco products are not missed during patient assessment.
  - These should be treated as a vital sign in the clinic setting, documented in the patient profile, and assessed periodically in the community pharmacy setting.
  - **Ask** About Tobacco Use
    - "Do you ever smoke or use any type of tobacco products?"
  - **Advise** to Quit
    - All patients who smoke should be advised to quit in a clear, strong, and personalized manner, using sensitivity in voice tone that communicates concern and willingness to assist the patient.
    - "I see you are now on two different inhalers for your COPD; quitting smoking is the single most important treatment to reduce your COPD symptoms and disease progression. I strongly encourage you to quit and would like to help you."
  - **Assess** Readiness to Quit
    - Patient should be categorized as (1) not ready to quit in the next month, (2) ready to quit in the next month, (3) recent quitter (≤6 months), (4) former user quitting 6 months ago or longer.
    - Counseling should be tailored to the patient's readiness.
    - "What are your thoughts about quitting? Is this something you may consider in the next month?"
  - **Assist** with Quitting
    - All patients ready to quit should be encouraged to use both behavioral counseling and pharmacotherapy, as combination provides greater likelihood of cessation than either alone.
      - Exception: Patients smoking less than 10 cigarettes/day
    - A quit date should be set within 1–2 weeks.

- **Arrange** Follow-Up Counseling
  - Follow-up should occur within 1 week of the quit date and a second within the first month. In-person or telephonic interventions can be used.

- The 5 R's Approach
  - Patients who aren't ready to quit should be encouraged to quit, and behavioral interventions should be used.
  - **Relevance**: information has a greater impact with personal meaning; encourage patients to think about why quitting is important to them.
  - **Risks**: ask patients to identify negative health consequences of smoking for themselves and others in their lives.
  - **Rewards**: work with patients to identify specific benefits of quitting.
  - **Roadblocks**: work with patients to help identify significant barriers to quitting and identify coping skills to address or circumvent each challenge.
  - **Repetition**: work with unsuccessful patients or patients who aren't yet motivated to identify triggers and repeat intervention steps.

■ ■ Qu**E**ST: Establish that the patient is an appropriate self-care candidate

Utilize the information collected in the patient assessment with the treatment algorithm and exclusions for self-care to determine if self-care is appropriate.

■ Exclusions to Self-Care

Review the treatment algorithm and exclusions for self-care provided at the beginning of the chapter. This section highlights key exclusion criteria.

■ Medications

- Current nicotine use—ideally, patients who smoke should not use NRT with other nicotine products; however, product labeling has changed to remove warnings against this as to not limit use in patients ready to try to quit.[2]

- Dual NRT use—labeling changes do not prohibit use of 2 types of NRT products together.[2] Combination therapy provides highest cessation rates.

- See Table 1 for a list of common drug interactions with tobacco smoke that should be considered in patients who successfully quit smoking.

TABLE 1. Relevant drug interactions with tobacco smoke for patients who quit

Drug, Class (Trade Name)	Mechanism of Interaction and Effects
Caffeine	Increased metabolism (induction of CYP1A2); increased clearance (56%). Caffeine levels are likely increased after cessation.
Clozapine (Clozaril)	Increased metabolism (induction of CYP1A2); decreased plasma concentrations (18%). Increased levels may occur upon cessation; closely monitor drug levels and reduce dose as required to avoid toxicity.
Erlotinib (Tarceva)	Increased clearance (24%); decreased trough serum concentrations (twofold) prior to quitting smoking.
Fluvoxamine (Luvox)	Increased metabolism (induction of CYP1A2); increased clearance (24%); decreased AUC (31%); decreased plasma concentrations (32%). Dosage modifications are not routinely recommended, but patient may require a decreased dose with successful cessation.
Haloperidol (Haldol)	Increased clearance (44%); decreased serum concentrations (70%) prior to quitting smoking
Methadone	Possible increased metabolism (induction of CYP1A2; minor pathway for methadone). Carefully monitor response upon cessation.
Olanzapine (Zyprexa)	Increased metabolism (induction of CYP1A2); increased clearance (98%). Dosage modifications are not routinely recommended, but patient may require a decreased dose with successful cessation.
Riociguat (Adempas)	Increased metabolism (induction of CYP1A1). Decreased plasma concentrations (by 50–60%). Patients who smoke may require dosages higher than 2.5 mg 3 times a day; consider dose reduction upon successful cessation.
Ropinirole (Requip)	Decreased maximum concentration (30%) and AUC (38%) in study with patients with restless legs syndrome. Patients may require a decreased dose with successful cessation.
Tacrine (Cognex)	Increased metabolism (induction of CYP1A2); decreased half-life (50%); serum concentrations threefold lower. Patients may require a decreased dose with successful cessation
Tasimelteon (Hetlioz)	Increased metabolism (induction of CYP1A2); drug exposure decreased by 40%. Patients may require a decreased dose with successful cessation.
Warfarin	Increased metabolism (induction of CYP1A2) of R-enantiomer; however, S-enantiomer is more potent, and the effect on the INR is inconclusive. Consider monitoring INR more closely upon smoking cessation.

Abbreviations used: AUC, area under the curve; INR, international normalized ratio.
Note: In most cases, the tobacco smoke—not the nicotine—causes these drug interactions. The majority of drug interactions are the result of induction of CYP P450 enzymes (primarily CYP1A2). The amount of tobacco smoking necessary to have an effect has not been established, and the assumption is that any smoker is susceptible to the same degree of interaction. Those exposed regularly to secondhand smoke may also be at risk.

⬛ Conditions

- NRT is only FDA-approved for cigarette smokers but is often used for smokeless tobacco users (e.g., chew, snuff). These patients should be referred to their health care providers.

- Serious heart disease (e.g., heart attack within 2 weeks, serious arrhythmias, serious or worsening angina)—should be evaluated for safety of NRT products before initiating.

- Uncontrolled hypertension—should have blood pressure control addressed while assessing appropriateness of NRT.

■ Special Populations

■ Pregnant and breastfeeding patients should be managed by their OB/GYN.

■ Adolescents less than 18 years of age should be referred to their health care provider as NRT products are only approved for those 18 years and older.

■ ■ QuE⑤T: Suggest appropriate self-care strategies

Select the appropriate treatment option based on the previously collected patient data. Various treatment options are discussed along with clinical pearls and pertinent patient considerations for optimal management.

■ Treatment Options

Consistent relief of withdrawal symptoms treatment of choice is the nicotine patch.

■ Nicotine Patches
   ▪ Patients should be started on the 21 mg/day patch for 4–6 weeks and slowly tapered to the 14 mg/day and 7 mg/day patches if the patient smokes 10 or more cigarettes/day. While the package labeling indicates starting with the 14 mg/day dose for patients who smoke less than 10 cigarettes/day, pharmacotherapy is not recommended in this patient population because of the lack of efficacy in enhancing likelihood of quitting smoking.
   ▪ Patients experiencing bothersome skin reactions can apply non-prescription hydrocortisone cream to the site or can use a different manufacturer's product with a different adhesive.
   ▪ Patients experiencing abnormal dreams can remove the patch at bedtime and apply a new patch upon waking.
   ▪ Patients experiencing dizziness, nausea, vomiting, diarrhea, headache, or perspiration should be changed to a lower dose.
   ▪ Adverse effects associated with nicotine patches include local skin reactions at the application site, abnormal dreams, insomnia, and headache. Nicotine absorption may cause slight redness, but allergic reactions will likely be raised or swollen, persist throughout use, and may have associated itching.

   > **CAUTIONS FOR NICOTINE PATCHES**
   > ▪ Patients with allergies to adhesive tape or skin problems (e.g., eczema, psoriasis, atopic dermatitis) should not use this product.

Acute nicotine withdrawal treatment of choice is nicotine polacrilex gum or nicotine polacrilex lozenge.

- Nicotine Polacrilex Gum and Lozenge
  - Nicotine polacrilex gum and lozenge provide immediate relief of nicotine withdrawal symptoms, and their dose is based on "time to first cigarette" (TTFC).
    - If TTFC is 30 minutes or less, the 4-mg dose should be used.
    - If TTFC is greater than 30 minutes, the 2-mg dose should be used.
  - The pharmacokinetics of the polacrilex lozenge offer ~25% more nicotine than an equivalent dose of gum because of complete dissolution of the dosage form.
  - Adverse effects associated with nicotine polacrilex gum and lozenge include unpleasant taste, mouth irritation, jaw soreness, dyspepsia, hiccups, and hypersalivation.

> **CAUTIONS FOR NICOTINE POLACRILEX GUM AND LOZENGE**
> - Patients with temporomandibular joint disease (TMJ) and teeth issues (e.g., dentures, braces) should not use nicotine gum.
> - The manufacturer recommends patients with diabetes and stomach ulcers contact their health care provider before using either product.

Other Treatment Considerations

- Optimal treatment would provide patients with a therapy to prevent withdrawal symptoms (patches, peak serum concentration in 3–12 hours) and a treatment for breakthrough cravings (gum, lozenge, peak serum concentration in 30–60 minutes).

- Nicotine patches may be preferred in patients who smoke continuously through the day because of a steady release of nicotine over 24 hours.

- Nicotine patches may be preferred in patients who struggle with taking multiple medication doses throughout the day.

- Nicotine gum and lozenges may be preferred in patients who want greater control in titrating nicotine levels to manage withdrawal symptoms.

- Nicotine gum and lozenges may be preferred in patients who smoke intermittently throughout the day or who smoke intensely in a short time frame.

- Complementary Therapy
  - Several herbal and homeopathic products are available for aid in cessation, but all lack data to support safety and efficacy.
  - *Lobelia inflata* is an herbal alkaloid with partial nicotinic agonist properties, but a meta-analysis and multicenter trial found no evidence to support use.
  - Acupuncture and hypnosis have not been found to be effective in clinical trials.
  - The United States Preventative Services Task Force (USPSTF) has concluded that current evidence available is insufficient to recommend e-cigarettes for tobacco cessation.[3] Patients should be discouraged from using e-cigarettes as a cessation tool, and use should be assessed as part of the patient workup.

Special Populations

- Pregnancy
  - NRT is classified by the FDA as Pregnancy Category D, although some experts have argued NRT is safer than continued smoking.

- Pediatric Patients
  - NRT is not approved for use in patients less than 18 years of age.

- Geriatric Patients
  - Patients 65 years of age and older can benefit greatly from quitting smoking, and there are no product limitations outside of comorbidities that may be seen in these patients.
  - If mobility is an issue, referral to a quit line may be helpful.

QuEST: Talk with the patient

Patient Education/Counseling

- Nonpharmacologic Talking Points
  - Apply the 5 A's approach with patients.
    - If the patient is not yet ready to quit, apply the 5 R's.
  - Refer the patient to 1-800-QUIT-NOW for behavioral counseling support.

- Tailor the session to the patient's needs, helping them remove triggers and develop approaches for withdrawal and cravings.

- Pharmacologic Talking Points
  - Nicotine Replacement Therapy
    - Patients should start NRT on the quit date and discontinue all forms of nicotine products upon initiation. There has been concern for nicotine-related adverse effects (e.g., nausea, palpitations) when patients continue to smoke while using NRT; however, patients who are motivated to quit should be met where they are.
    - Patients should be advised that NRT products provide less nicotine than combustible cigarettes and thus won't feel "as good" as smoking a cigarette.
    - Nicotine Patch
      - Apply to a clean, dry, hairless area of the skin on the upper body or upper outer part of the arm at the same time every day, rotating location each day. The same location should not be used more than once a week to minimize irritation.
      - Apply firm pressure with the palm of the hand for 10 seconds, including the edges for a good seal.
      - Wash hands after applying or removing a patch.
      - Leftover adhesive can be removed with rubbing alcohol.
      - Do not cut patches—nicotine may evaporate from cut edges.
      - The patch should be removed before magnetic resonance imaging (MRI) procedures.
      - Discard by folding onto itself, completely covering adhesive area
    - Polacrilex Gum
      - Patients should be counseled to chew differently than regular gum, using the "chew and park" approach—chewing until a peppery or tingling sensation, parking gum between the cheek and buccal area until that sensation goes away, then chewing again. When peppery taste returns, park in a different location to avoid mouth irritation.
      - Chewing gum too rapidly can cause excessive release of nicotine, worsening adverse effects.
      - Each piece of gum should last ~30 minutes.

- To minimize withdrawal symptoms, use on a scheduled basis rather than as needed. Initial use of every 1–2 hours requires a minimum of 9 pieces a day for greatest effectiveness.
- Food and beverages should not be consumed for 15 minutes before and while using the gum.
  □ Polacrilex Lozenge
  - Place the lozenge in the mouth and allow it to slowly dissolve (~20–30 minutes).
  - Occasionally rotate to different areas of the mouth to decrease mouth irritation.
  - Heartburn and indigestion are likely if the lozenge is chewed, swallowed, multiple are used together, or one is used right after another; thus, these strategies should be avoided.
  - To minimize withdrawal symptoms, use on a scheduled basis rather than as needed. Initial use of every 1–2 hours requires a minimum of 9 lozenges a day for greatest effectiveness.
  - Food and beverages should not be consumed for 15 minutes before and while using the lozenge.

- Suggest medical referral if any of the following occur:
  - Serious cardiovascular symptoms (e.g., palpitations)
  - Symptoms of nicotine overdose (e.g., nausea, vomiting, diarrhea, dizziness, weakness)
  - Symptoms of irritation (e.g., mouth soreness, tooth soreness, severe sore throat, persistent indigestion) with gum or lozenge products

Clinical Pearls

- Smoking causes induction of the CYP1A2 isoenzyme, increasing the hepatic metabolism of substrates and potentially resulting in decreased therapeutic response or increased dosages. Dosages of CYP1A2-affected medications may need to be reduced in patients who quit smoking. Similarly, the clearance of caffeine is significantly increased; when quitting, patients who smoke and drink caffeinated beverages should be advised to decrease their usual caffeine intake to avoid symptoms similar to nicotine withdrawal.

- The most effective therapies are prescription-only varenicline and combination nicotine patches with as-needed NRT. Ideally, the Ask-Advise-Refer model should be utilized for patients who are ready to quit and referred to a health care provider for prescription therapy or more extensive counseling.

■ ● References

1. Martin BA, Wopat MC. Tobacco cessation. In: Krinsky DL, Ferreri SP, Hemstreet BA, Hume AL, Newton GD, Rollins CJ, Tietze KJ, eds. *Handbook of Nonprescription Drugs: An Interactive Approach to Self-Care*. Washington, DC: American Pharmacists Association; 2017:873–898.

2. U.S. Food and Drug Administration. Nicotine replacement therapy labels may change. https://www.integration.samhsa.gov/health-wellness/NRT_Label_Change_0413.pdf. Accessed October 1, 2017.

3. Patnode CD, Henderson JT, Thompson JH, et al. Behavioral counseling and pharmaco-therapy interventions for tobacco cessation in adults, including pregnant women: A review of reviews for the U.S. Preventative Services Task Force. *Ann Intern Med.* 2015;163(8):608–621.

WARTS

Karen Steinmetz Pater, PharmD, CDE, BCACP

For complete information about this topic, consult Chapter 43, "Warts," written by Donna M. Adkins and published in the *Handbook of Nonprescription Drugs*, 19th edition.[1]

Self-Care of Warts

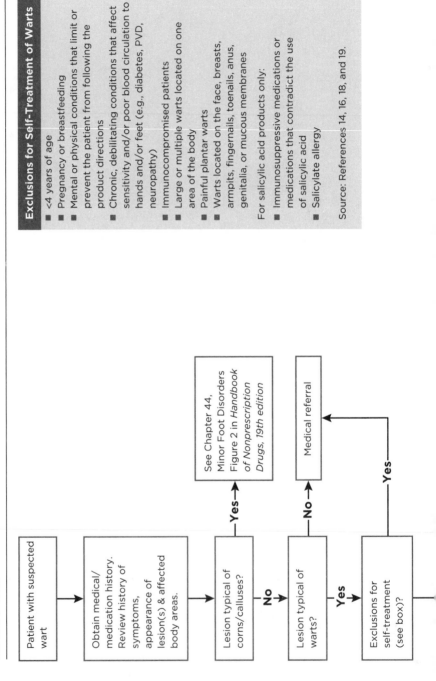

Exclusions for Self-Treatment of Warts

- <4 years of age
- Pregnancy or breastfeeding
- Mental or physical conditions that limit or prevent the patient from following the product directions
- Chronic, debilitating conditions that affect sensitivity and/or poor blood circulation to hands and/or feet (e.g., diabetes, PVD, neuropathy)
- Immunocompromised patients
- Large or multiple warts located on one area of the body
- Painful plantar warts
- Warts located on the face, breasts, armpits, fingernails, toenails, anus, genitalia, or mucous membranes

For salicylic acid products only:

- Immunosuppressive medications or medications that contradict the use of salicylic acid
- Salicylate allergy

Source: References 14, 16, 18, and 19.

Patient with suspected wart

↓

Obtain medical/medication history. Review history of symptoms, appearance of lesion(s) & affected body areas.

↓

Lesion typical of corns/calluses? —**Yes**→ See Chapter 44, Minor Foot Disorders Figure 2 in *Handbook of Nonprescription Drugs, 19th edition*

↓ **No**

Lesion typical of warts? —**No**→ Medical referral

↓ **Yes**

Exclusions for self-treatment (see box)? —**Yes**→ (to Medical referral)

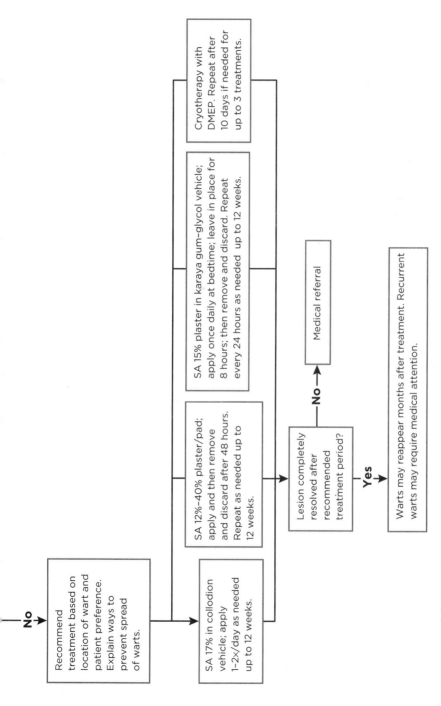

Recommend treatment based on location of wart and patient preference. Explain ways to prevent spread of warts.

No

SA 17% in collodion vehicle; apply 1–2×/day as needed up to 12 weeks.

SA 12%–40% plaster/pad; apply and then remove and discard after 48 hours. Repeat as needed up to 12 weeks.

SA 15% plaster in karaya gum–glycol vehicle; apply once daily at bedtime; leave in place for 8 hours; then remove and discard. Repeat every 24 hours as needed up to 12 weeks.

Cryotherapy with DMEP. Repeat after 10 days if needed for up to 3 treatments.

Lesion completely resolved after recommended treatment period?

No → Medical referral

Yes → Warts may reappear months after treatment. Recurrent warts may require medical attention.

DMEP = Dimethyl ether and propane; PVD = peripheral vascular disease; SA = salicylic acid.

■ ● Overview

■ Warts, also known as verrucae, are a common skin disorder caused by human papillomaviruses (HPVs).

■ Warts are benign conditions that often go away without treatment. There is no cure for HPV infection.

■ The goal of self-treatment is to eliminate signs and symptoms associated with warts, remove warts without causing scars, and prevent transmission to others or other locations of the body.

■ ● Pathophysiology

■ HPV infection is limited to the epidermal tissues and does not spread systemically.

■ HPV may enter the epidermal layer of the skin and infect the basal keratinocytes when minor skin abrasions are present.

■ Warts may affect skin and mucous membranes anywhere on the body. HPV-2, HPV-4, HPV-27, and HPV-57 are the most common causes of warts on the hands, and HPV-1 is the most common cause of warts on the feet.

■ The incubation period of HPV may be months, with the manifestation of warts possibly dependent on the immune response of the infected individual.

● Transmission

■ HPV infection occurs via person-to-person contact, autoinoculation, or contact with fomites on contaminated surfaces.

● Preventative Measures

■ To decrease the chance of getting warts, avoid nail-biting, do not go barefoot (especially on wet surfaces), and keep feet clean and dry. Swimming pools and public showers can increase risk of transmission.

■ To avoid spreading warts from one part of your body to another, do not cut, shave, or pick at warts; wash hands before and after treating or touching warts; use one specific towel to dry warts; and do not use the same towel to dry other areas of the body.

■ To avoid spreading warts to others, do not share towels, razors, socks, shoes, etc.; keep the wart covered; and do not walk barefoot.

■ ■ ⒬EST: Quickly and Accurate Assess the Patient Using SCHOLAR MAC

QuEST SCHOLAR is an acronym used to assess a patient to determine self-care candidate status and to identify which treatment would be most appropriate. See Chapter 1 for a description of the QuEST SCHOLAR process.

■ Does the Patient Have Common Warts?

■ Presence of skin-colored or brown, hyperkeratotic, dome-shaped papules with rough cauliflower-like appearance

■ Frequently found on the hands

■ Generally not associated with pain

■ Does the Patient Have Plantar Warts?

■ Presence of skin-colored callous-like lesions on the feet; generally affects a larger surface area than seen on the hands

■ Can be associated with pain, especially if occurring in a weight-bearing location

■ Important SCHOLAR MAC Considerations

■ Where is the location of the warts?
  ■ The FDA recommends self-treatment of warts be limited to common and plantar warts.
  ■ The appropriate concentration of salicylic acid (SA) will differ between common and plantar warts.

■ If papules are present on the foot, where are they located?
  ■ If located over bony prominences or on weight-bearing areas, may be a corn or callus and not a wart

■ Is the lesion bleeding?
  ■ Bleeding may be a sign of a malignant growth; medical referral is necessary.

■ Are the lesions associated with friction or accompanying skin abrasions?
  ■ Skin abrasions may serve as an entry point for HPV, the cause of warts.
  ■ Friction is typically the causative factor of corns and calluses.

■ See Table 1 for differentiation of warts and skin disorders with similar presentations.

● *Physical Assessment Techniques*

■ Common Warts
- ▪ Observe the hands for number, size, and location of the warts.

■ Plantar Warts
- ▪ Observe the foot for singular wart versus clustering of warts (called mosaic wart), which is generally viewed as one large wart.
- ▪ Observe the patient while walking to determine if gait is affected by pain associated with the wart.

TABLE 1. Differentiation of warts and skin disorders with similar presentation

Criterion	Warts	Corns	Calluses	Malignant Growth
Location	Any area of skin susceptible to the virus	Over bony prominences in the feet	Weight-bearing areas of the feet	Any area of the skin
Signs	Rough cauliflower-like appearance; plantar warts disrupt normal skin ridges	Raised, sharply demarcated, hyperkeratotic lesions with a central core	Raised yellowish thickening of the skin; broad-based with diffuse borders; normal pattern of skin ridges	Bleeding; swelling; red, discolored, or multicolored
Symptoms	Usually not painful, but pain may occur if the wart is located in areas undergoing repeated pressure (e.g., soles of the feet)	Pain	Usually not painful, but pain may occur if the callus is located in an area where significant pressure may occur (e.g., soles of the feet)	Pain
Quantity, severity	Varies; may grow to approximately 1 in in diameter	Varies; a few millimeters to 1 cm	Varies; a few millimeters to several centimeters	Varies; grows rapidly
Timing	Incubation period may be several months; may progressively enlarge	Variable onset; may progressively enlarge	Variable onset; may progressively enlarge	Variable onset; grows rapidly
Cause	HPV infection of the epidermal layer	Friction	Friction, walking barefoot, structural foot problems	Mutations related to damaged DNA cause skin cells to grow unchecked
Modifying factors	Prevention of spread; treatment with SA or cryotherapy	Alleviation of causative factors; treatment with SA	Alleviation of causative factors; treatment with SA	Surgical removal; prescription medications

■ ■ Qu🅔ST: Establish that the patient is an appropriate self-care candidate

Utilize the information collected in the patient assessment with the treatment algorithm and exclusions for self-care to determine if self-care is appropriate.

■ Exclusions to Self-Care

Review the treatment algorithm and exclusions for self-care provided at the beginning of the chapter. This section highlights key exclusion criteria.

■ Medications

■ Immunosuppressive medications—warts are less likely to resolve spontaneously in adults who are immunocompromised. Wait-and-see approach is not appropriate.

■ Conditions

■ Chronic conditions that affect sensitivity or circulation of the hands or feet, such as diabetes, peripheral vascular disease, or neuropathy, require a different treatment approach. Patients with these conditions may have delayed healing time for wounds, and SA could further impede wound healing or promote further injury.

■ Immunocompromising conditions (e.g., rheumatoid arthritis, systemic lupus erythematous) make warts less likely to heal spontaneously. Wait-and-see is likely not appropriate, and drug therapy should be initiated.

■ Special Populations

■ Children under 4 years of age should be referred to their pediatrician because of the risk of systemic absorption of therapy and potential for damage to the young child's skin.

■ SA should not be used in children less than 16 years of age with viral illnesses because of the risk of Reye's syndrome.

■ Frail older adults may not be appropriate candidates for self-care because of thinner, more friable skin. Special care to avoid treatment to normal skin is essential.

■ ■ QuE⑤T: Suggest appropriate self-care strategies

Select the appropriate treatment option based on the previously collected patient data. Various treatment options are discussed along with clinical pearls and pertinent patient considerations for optimal management.

■ Treatment Options

Common and plantar warts treatment of choice is SA or dimethyl ether and propane (DMEP).

- ■ Salicylic Acid
  - ▪ SA and DMEP appear to be equally effective, so product selection is based on patient preference.
  - ▪ SA is available in a variety of formulations:
    - □ SA 17% should be used for common warts.
    - □ SA 40% or higher should be used for plantar warts.
  - ▪ Self-treatment with SA should not continue past 12 weeks.
  - ▪ Adverse effects associated with SA include skin irritation and potential for systemic toxicity.

> **CAUTIONS FOR SA**
>
> - ▪ There is potential to damage healthy skin surrounding the wart. Treatment should be applied directly on the wart, and application to noninfected tissues should be avoided.
> - ▪ Suggest protecting adjacent healthy skin from coming into contact with SA.

- ■ Cryotherapy with Dimethyl Ether and Propane
  - ▪ A blister will form under the wart, and the wart will fall off after about 10 days.
  - ▪ Treatment may be repeated every 2 weeks if necessary for a maximum of 4 treatments over 12 weeks. Treating every 2–3 weeks yields the best results.
  - ▪ Adverse effects associated with DMEP include pain, blistering, scarring, hypo- or hyperpigmentation, and tendon or nerve damage with aggressive therapy.

> **CAUTIONS FOR CRYOTHERAPY**
> - Patients must follow directions on the label carefully to avoid damaging healthy skin surrounding the wart.
> - Avoid using the applicators more than once to avoid reinfecting the tissue or spreading the virus to others.

Other Treatment Considerations

- A wait-and-see approach without nonprescription treatment is also an option, but it allows for the continued spread of warts through auto-inoculation and transmission to others.
- The use of duct tape as an occlusive aid for clearance of warts has become a popular, inexpensive treatment option.
- Two randomized controlled trials evaluating the use of duct tape for clearance of warts are available, one in favor of duct tape and one with conflicting results. More evidence is needed before widespread use of duct tape as a definitive treatment can be suggested, although it may have a place in therapy for small children with warts.

Complementary Therapy

- Vitamin A (retinoids) may interfere with HPV replication; a case report showed improvement in recalcitrant warts after 6 months of treatment, but data are weak.
- Dietary zinc is hypothesized to improve immune response and inhibit HPV replication; limited data show benefit in recalcitrant warts.
- Garlic is thought to inhibit proliferation of virus-infected cells. Application of chloroform extracts resulted in complete resolution after 1–2 weeks, and there was no reoccurrence after 3–4 months.
- All data for complementary therapy are limited and cannot be extrapolated to a population at large. Use is likely best with SA or DMEP for recalcitrant warts.

Special Populations

Pregnancy

- The effects of topical SA and cryotherapy with DMEP on an unborn child are not known. Because of the risk for systemic absorption, these products should not be used for self-treatment in pregnancy.

- Patients who are pregnant should be referred to their obstetrician or primary care provider for treatment of warts.
- Breastfeeding
    - It is unknown if topical SA passes into breast milk in sufficient amounts to harm a nursing infant. Use of products containing SA is not recommended in patients who are lactating; however, if the patient wishes to self-treat warts with these products, they should discontinue nursing for the duration of use.
    - It is unknown how cryotherapy with DMEP affects an infant who is breastfeeding, and use in patients who are lactating is not recommended.
- Pediatric Patients
    - SA use should be approved by a pediatrician because of risk for skin damage and Reye's syndrome if the child had a concomitant viral illness.
    - It is unknown how cryotherapy with DMEP may affect the skin of young children, and use in children younger than 4 years of age is not recommended.
- Geriatric Patients
    - Older healthy adults may use both SA-containing products and cryotherapy with DMEP in a manner similar to that in younger adults.
    - Care should be taken to avoid damaging the normal skin tissue around the wart when using these products.

⬛ ⬤ QuES⬤: Talk with the patient

⬛ Patient Education/Counseling

- Nonpharmacologic Talking Points
    - If duct tape is used, it should be applied for a prolonged time (~6 days) and then replaced.
    - Wart Removal Preparation
        - Wash hands before and after use.
        - Soak the affected area for 5 minutes.
        - Wash and dry the affected area thoroughly.
        - May use a file or pumice stone to lightly remove the surface of plantar warts
- Pharmacologic Talking Points
    - Salicylic Acid
        - Keep these products away from the eyes.
        - Do not use to treat warts on the face, mucous membranes, armpits, breasts, genitals, or around the nail beds.

- If these products come into contact with healthy skin, wash the area with soap and water immediately.
- Improvement should be seen within 1–2 weeks of starting treatment. The wart should completely clear within 6–12 weeks.
- Products are flammable; keep away from heat sources.

- Cryotherapy with DMEP
  - Do not use to treat warts on the face, mucous membranes, armpits, breasts, genitals, or around the nail beds.
  - Patients will feel an aching, stinging sensation when the product is applied.
  - Patients should apply DMEP directly to the wart and limit contact with normal skin.
  - Do not use this product if patients cannot follow instructions directly as written. Each product will have similar application instructions, but product-specific application directions exist.
  - Products are flammable; keep away from heat sources.

- Suggest medical referral if any of the following occur:
  - SA products come into contact with the eyes
  - Severe irritation or pain immediately following application of either treatment
  - Frequent recurrence of warts after treatment
  - Patients should start to see improvement in 1–2 weeks. Follow-up with the healthcare provider should occur after 4–6 weeks to evaluate the wart. If it has not cleared by 12 weeks, prescription therapies may be warranted.

Clinical Pearls

- Patients with multiple warts, warts on the fingernails, or large warts should be evaluated by a primary care provider.

- Application of skin protectants (e.g., Vaseline, white petrolatum) may be considered around the wart on healthy tissue to prevent damage of normal skin.

References

1. Adkins D. Warts. In: Krinsky DL, Ferreri SP, Hemstreet BA, Hume AL, Newton GD, Rollins CJ, Tietze KJ, eds. *Handbook of Nonprescription Drugs: An Interactive Approach to Self-Care*. Washington, DC: American Pharmacists Association; 2017:809–820.

Administration Guidelines for Nasal, Ophthalmic, and Otic Dosage Formulations

Jennifer A. Wilson, PharmD, BCACP
and Rashi Chandra Waghel, PharmD, BCACP

For complete information about this topic, consult Chapter 11, "Colds and Allergy," written by Kelly L. Scolaro; Chapter 28, "Ophthalmic Disorders," written by Richard G. Fiscella and Michael K. Jensen; and Chapter 30, "Otic Disorders," written by Veronica T. Bandy and published in the *Handbook of Nonprescription Drugs*, 19th Edition.[1-3]

■ ● Nasal Dosage Formulations

Administration Guidelines for Nasal Dosage Formulations

General Instructions

- Clear nasal passages before administering the product.
- Wash your hands before and after use.
- Gently depress the other side of the nose with finger to close off the nostril not receiving the medication.
- Aim tip of delivery device **away** from nasal septum to avoid accidental damage to the septum.
- Breathe through mouth and wait a few minutes after using the medication before blowing the nose.

Nasal Sprays

- Gently insert the bottle tip into one nostril, as shown in drawing A.
- Keep head upright. Sniff deeply while squeezing the bottle. Repeat with other nostril.

Nasal Inhalers

- Warm the inhaler in hand just before use.
- Gently insert the inhaler tip into one nostril, as shown in drawing C. Sniff deeply while inhaling.
- Wipe the inhaler after each use. Discard after 2–3 months even if the inhaler still smells medicinal.

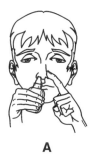

A

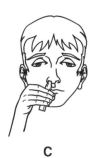

C

Pump Nasal Sprays

- Prime the pump before using it the first time. Hold the bottle with the nozzle placed between the first two fingers and the thumb placed on the bottom of the bottle.
- Tilt the head forward.
- Gently insert the nozzle tip into one nostril, as shown in drawing B. Sniff deeply while depressing the pump once.
- Repeat with other nostril.

Nasal Drops

- Lie on bed with head tilted back and over the side of the bed, as shown in drawing D.
- Squeeze the bulb to withdraw medication from the bottle.
- Place the recommended number of drops into one nostril. Gently tilt head from side to side.
- Repeat with other nostril. Lie on bed for a couple of minutes after placing drops in the nose.
- Do not rinse the dropper.

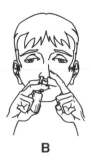

B

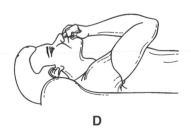

D

Note: Do not share the drug with anyone. Discard solutions if discolored or if contamination is suspected. Remove caps before use and replace tightly after each use. Do not use expired products.

■ ■ Ophthalmic Dosage Formulations

Administration Guidelines for Eyedrops

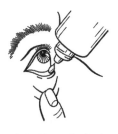

1. If you have difficulty determining whether eyedrops have been successfully instilled into your eye, refrigerate the solution before administering it—the cold drops on the eye surface are easily detected. Do not refrigerate suspensions, however. Always check the expiration date.
2. Wash hands thoroughly. Wash areas of the face around the eyes. Contact lenses should be removed unless the product is designed specifically for use with contact lenses.
3. Tilt head back. When administering drops to children, have the patient lie down before placing drops in the eyes.
4. Gently grasp lower outer eyelid below lashes, and pull eyelid away from eye to create a pouch.
5. Place dropper over eye by looking directly at it, as shown in the drawing.
6. Just before applying a single drop, look up.
7. As soon as the drop is applied, release the eyelid slowly. Close eyes gently for 3 minutes and position the head downward as though looking at the floor (using gravity to pull the drop onto the cornea). Minimize blinking or squeezing of the eyelid.
8. Use a finger to put gentle pressure over the opening of the tear duct.
9. Blot excessive solution from around the eye.
10. If multiple medications are indicated, wait at least 5 minutes before instilling the next drop. This pause helps ensure that the first drop is not flushed away by the second and that the second drop is not diluted by the first.
11. If using a suspension, shake well before instilling. If using the suspension with another dosage form, place the suspension drop last, because it has prolonged retention time in the tear film.
12. If both drop and ointment therapy are indicated, instill the drops at least 10 minutes before the ointment so that the ointment does not present a barrier to the drops' penetration of the tear film or cornea.

Administration Guidelines for Eye Ointments

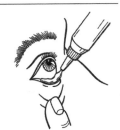

1. Wash hands thoroughly. Wash areas of the face around the eyes.
2. If both drop and ointment therapy are indicated, instill the drops at least 10 minutes before the ointment so that the ointment does not present a barrier to the drops' penetration of the tear film or cornea.
3. Tilt head back.
4. Gently grasp lower outer eyelid below lashes, and pull eyelid away from eye, as shown in the drawing.
5. Place ointment tube over eye by looking directly at it.
6. With a sweeping motion, place a strip of ointment, one-fourth to one-half inch wide, inside the lower eyelid by gently squeezing the tube, but avoid touching the tube tip to any tissue surface.
7. Release the eyelid slowly.
8. Close eyes gently for 1–2 minutes.
9. Blot excessive ointment from around the eye.
10. Vision may be blurred temporarily. Avoid activities that require good visual ability until vision clears.

■■ Otic Dosage Formulations

Guidelines for Administering Eardrops

1. Wash your hands with soap and warm water; then dry them thoroughly.
2. Carefully wash and dry the outside of the ear with a damp washcloth, taking care not to get water in the ear canal. Then dry the ear.
3. Warm eardrops to body temperature by holding the container in the palm of your hand for a few minutes. Do not warm the container in hot water or microwave. Instilling hot eardrops can cause ear pain, nausea, or dizziness.
4. If the label indicates, gently shake the container to mix contents.
5. Tilt your head (or have the patient tilt the head) to the side, as shown in drawing A. Or lie down with the affected ear up, as shown in drawing B. Use gentle restraint, if necessary, for an infant or a young child.
6. Open the container carefully. Position the dropper tip near, but not inside, the ear canal opening. Do not allow the dropper to touch the ear, because it could become contaminated or injure the ear. Eardrop bottles must be kept clean.
7. Pull your ear (or the patient's ear) backward and upward to open the ear canal (drawing A). If the patient is a child younger than 3 years, pull the ear backward and downward (drawing B).
8. Place the proper dose or number of drops into the ear canal. Replace the cap on the container.
9. Gently press the small, flat skin flap (tragus) over the ear canal opening to force out air bubbles and push the drops down the ear canal.
10. Stay (or keep the patient) in the same position for the length of time indicated in the product instructions. If the patient is a child who cannot stay still, the primary care provider may tell you to place a clean piece of cotton gently into the child's ear to prevent the medication from draining out. Use a piece large enough to remove easily, and do not leave it in the ear longer than 1 hour.
11. Repeat the procedure for the other ear, if needed.
12. Gently wipe excess medication off the outside of the ear, using caution to avoid getting moisture in the ear canal.
13. Wash your hands to remove any medication.

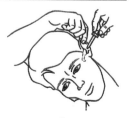

A

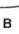

B

Source: *APhA Special Report: Medication Administration Problem Solving in Ambulatory Care.* Washington, DC: American Pharmaceutical Association; 1994:9.

Guidelines for Removing Excessive or Impacted Cerumen

Ceruminolytics

1. Place 5–10 drops of the cerumen-softening solution into the ear canal, and allow it to remain for at least 15 minutes, as described in Table 30–1.
2. Perform this procedure daily for no longer than 4 consecutive days.

Irrigation Technique

The use of ceruminolytics and irrigation together may improve overall removal of impacted cerumen. The ceruminolytic agent is administered first. Then follow the irrigation technique as described below, paying special attention to cautionary instructions.

1. Prepare a warm (not hot) solution of plain water or other solution as directed by your primary care provider. Eight ounces of solution should be sufficient to clean out the ear canal.
2. To catch the returning solution, hold a container under the ear being cleaned. An emesis basin is ideal because it fits the contour of the neck. Tilt the head slightly toward the side of the ear being cleaned.
3. Gently pull the earlobe down and back to expose the ear canal, as shown in drawing A.
4. Place the open end of the syringe into the ear canal with the tip pointed slightly upward toward the side of the ear canal (drawing A). Do not aim the syringe to the back of the ear canal. Make sure that the syringe does not obstruct the outflow of solution.
5. Squeeze the bulb gently—not forcefully—to introduce the solution into the ear canal and to avoid rupturing the eardrum. (Note: Only health care professionals trained in aural hygiene should use forced water spray irrigators [e.g., Waterpik] to remove cerumen.)
6. Do not let the returning solution come into contact with the eyes.
7. If pain or dizziness occurs, remove the syringe and do not resume irrigation until a health care provider is consulted.
8. Make sure all water is drained from the ear to avoid predisposing to infection from presence of excessive moisture (water-clogged ears).
9. Rinse the syringe thoroughly before and after each use, and let it dry.
10. Store the syringe in a cool, dry place (preferably, in its original container) away from hot surfaces and sharp instruments
11. If cerumen still remains, consult your primary care provider.

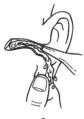

A

Source: Adapted with permission from *Ohio Clin.* 1996;14(5):10.

■■ References

1. Scolaro KL. Colds and allergy. In: Krinsky DL, Ferreri SP, Henstreet BA, Hume AL, Newton GD, Rollins CJ, Tietze KJ, eds. *Handbook of Nonprescription Drugs: An Interactive Approach to Self-Care.* Washington, DC: American Pharmacists Association; 2017:192.

2. Fiscella RG and Jensen MK. Ophthalmic disorders. In: Krinsky DL, Ferreri SP, Henstreet BA, Hume AL, Newton GD, Rollins CJ, Tietze KJ, eds. *Handbook of Nonprescription Drugs: An Interactive Approach to Self-Care.* Washington, DC: American Pharmacists Association; 2017:550.

3. Bandy VT. Otic disorders. In: Krinsky DL, Ferreri SP, Henstreet BA, Hume AL, Newton GD, Rollins CJ, Tietze KJ. *Handbook of Nonprescription Drugs: An Interactive Approach to Self-Care.* Washington, DC: American Pharmacists Association; 2017:594–595.

Guidelines for Temperature Measurement

Connie Kang, PharmD, BCPS, BCGP

For complete information about this topic, consult Chapter 6, "Fever," written by Virginia Lemay and Brett Feret and published in the *Handbook of Nonprescription Drugs*, 19th Edition.[1]

■ ● General Temperature Measurement Guidelines

■ Over the course of an illness, measure body temperature with the same thermometer at the same anatomical site, because readings from different thermometers or sites may vary. Further information in addition to what is provided in this appendix is available in the "Fever" chapter.

■ Estimates of core temperature measured at different anatomical sites may vary in terms of what is considered elevated. On average, the following temperatures represent a fever for the following sites of measurement:
- **Rectal** temperature greater than 100.4°F (38.0°C)
- **Oral** temperature greater than 99.5°F (37.5°C)
- **Axillary** temperature greater than 99.3°F (37.4°C)
- **Tympanic** temperature greater than 100.0°F (37.8°C)
- **Temporal** measurement greater than 100.1°F (37.8°C) for **over 4 years** of age
- **Temporal** measurement greater than 100.3°F (37.9°C) for **3–47 months** of age
- **Temporal** measurement greater than 100.7°F (38.1°C) for **0–2 months** of age

■ Site(s) of temperature measurement by age:
- **Younger than 3 months** of age: **rectal** method of temperature measurement is preferred if caregiver can safely use this route.
- **3 months–3 years** of age: **rectal, oral,** or **temporal** method of temperature measurement may be used.
- **Tympanic** method of temperature measurement may be used starting at **6 months** of age.
- **Older than 3 years** of age: **oral, tympanic,** or **temporal** method of temperature measurement is appropriate.

■ Patient-related factors may preclude the use of a particular type of thermometer (e.g., diarrhea or hemorrhoids are relative contraindications for use of a rectal thermometer).

■ When assessing patient fevers, it is important to know if the fever has been treated (e.g., medication, dose, administration time).

■ Instruct caregivers or patients to keep a timed log that may include temperatures, sites of measurement, and medications with doses.

■ The U.S. Food and Drug Administration regulates thermometers as medical devices; all approved types of thermometers are accurate and reliable if used appropriately.

■ ■ Guidelines for Temperature Measurement Using Electronic Thermometers

■ *Rectal*

- Gold standard because it is the closest estimate of core temperature

- While potentially intrusive, appropriate for use in most patients of all ages (preferred in infants up to 3 months of age)

- Readings in approximately 10–60 seconds

- A thermometer that is used rectally should not be used subsequently for oral measurement.

- Patients should never be unattended while rectal thermometer remains in place.

- Slow to detect rapid changes in body temperature because of poor blood flow within large muscle mass

1. Place clean probe cover over tip.
2. Turn on and wait until it indicates it is ready for use.
3. Apply a water-soluble lubricant to thermometer tip.
4. *For infants or young children*, place child facedown over caregiver's lap, separate the buttocks with the thumb and forefinger of one hand, and insert gently in the direction of the child's umbilicus. *For infants*, insert to the length of the tip only. *For young children*, insert about 1 in. For safety, hold the thermometer at these age-appropriate distances and insert the tip until the finger touches the anus.
5. *For adults*, lie on one side with the legs flexed to approximately a 45-degree angle from the abdomen. Insert the tip 0.5–2 in by holding the thermometer 0.5–2 in away from the tip and inserting it until the finger touches the anus. Have the patient take a deep breath during this process to facilitate proper positioning of the thermometer.
6. Hold the thermometer in place until it beeps and temperature is displayed.
7. Remove thermometer and record the temperature.
8. Dispose of probe cover and clean thermometer with an antiseptic (e.g., alcohol, povidone-iodine solution) by wiping away from the stem toward tip. Rinse with cool water.
9. Wipe any remaining lubricant from the anus.

Oral

- Oral probe thermometers may not be ideal for most children under 3 years of age because of difficulties with placement and a tight seal; pacifier thermometers may be recommended instead of oral probe thermometers in infants and children between 3 months and 3 years of age.

- Oral temperature should not be obtained in a patient who is mouth breathing or hyperventilating, is not fully alert, or is uncooperative, lethargic, or confused.

- Readings in approximately 10–60 seconds

ORAL PROBE

1. Wait 20–30 minutes after drinking or eating.
2. Place a clean disposable probe cover over tip.
3. Turn on thermometer and wait until it is ready for use.
4. Place tip under tongue.
5. Close mouth and breathe through nose.
6. Hold thermometer in place until it beeps.
7. Remove thermometer from mouth and record the displayed temperature.
8. Remove and dispose of probe cover.
9. Disinfect if thermometer is a shared device for multiple users.

ORAL PACIFIER

1. Wait 30 minutes after drinking or eating.
2. Inspect the pacifier for any tears or cracks. Do not use if worn.
3. Press the button to turn on.
4. Place pacifier in child's mouth.
5. Have child hold pacifier in mouth without moving, if possible, for time specified on thermometer packaging.
6. Remove thermometer after the beep and record the temperature.

Axillary

- Relatively noninvasive; however, it is less reliable than oral and rectal methods. If fever is detected, recommend confirming with an alternative method

- Do not measure immediately after bathing or vigorous activity, which can temporarily affect body temperature without elevating the thermoregulatory set point.

- Readings in approximately 10–60 seconds

1. Place clean disposable probe cover over tip.
2. Turn on and wait until it is ready for use.
3. Place tip in clean and dry armpit. Thermometer must be touching skin, not clothing.
4. Ensure tight seal and avoid arm movement. If taking a child's temperature, hold child close to secure thermometer within child's armpit, if necessary.
5. Read and record temperature when thermometer beeps.

■ ● Guidelines for Temperature Measurement Using Infrared Thermometers

● *Tympanic*

■ Noninvasive; however, requires infrared measurement specifically from the tympanic membrane

■ Accuracy of reading can be affected by several factors including positioning, ear wax, and ear infection

■ May be more accurate than axillary or oral temperatures in estimating core temperature when used appropriately

■ Not recommended in infants less than 6 months of age because of inaccurate readings that are due to ear canals not being fully developed.

■ Extremely quick readings (<5 seconds), which can help with measurement in young children

1. Place a clean disposable lens cover over ear probe.
2. Turn on thermometer and wait until it is ready for use.
3. For children *younger than 1 year* of age, pull ear backward to straighten ear canal. Place ear probe into canal and aim the tip of the probe toward patient's eye.
4. For patients *older than 1 year* of age, pull ear backward and up to straighten ear canal. Place the ear probe into canal and aim the tip of probe toward patient's eye.
5. Press the button for temperature measurement.
6. Read and record temperature when device beeps.
7. Discard lens cover.

■ ■ Temporal Touch

- ■ Extremely quick (<5 seconds) and noninvasive nature makes the temporal thermometer a preferable route for most patients.

- ■ More sensitive to fever detection than tympanic measurements in infants, but the temporal thermometer has not shown superiority over the rectal method.

- ■ Presence of hair may affect accuracy of reading.

- ■ Newer no-touch infrared thermometers (temporal or alternate sites) have the benefit of not having to wake a child; however, they are less reliable and accurate than rectal method in children.

1. Allow thermometer to acclimatize to the environment for about 30 minutes if the thermometer was moved from a hot room to a cold room or vice versa.
2. Move hair away from the temples, forehead, and behind the earlobe.
3. Place probe on one side of forehead (near temporal area).
4. Depress button and hold while scanning for the temporal artery temperature.
5. Sweep thermometer across forehead to the hairline on the opposite side of the head. Ensure probe remains in contact with skin at all times and hold button down until finished scanning.
6. If there is sweat on the forehead, sweep the thermometer as normal, but nestle the thermometer on the neck directly behind the earlobe before releasing the button.
7. Lift thermometer, release the button, and record the temperature.

■ ■ References

1. Lemay V, Feret B. Fever. In: Krinksy DL, Ferreri SP, Hemstreet BA, Hume AL, Newton GD, Rollins CJ, Tietze KJ, eds. *Handbook of Nonprescription Drugs: An Interactive Approach to Self-Care.* Washington, DC: American Pharmacists Association; 2017:97–110.

FDA Pregnancy Risk Categories

Albert Bach, PharmD

- The decision to use drugs during pregnancy ultimately lies in the assessment of the risk-benefit ratio between the woman and her health care providers.

- The Food and Drug Administration (FDA) has established guidelines that provide patients and health care providers with the available evidence for a drug's use in pregnant women. In 2014, the FDA published new requirements for communicating pregnancy and lactation risks for drugs in a final rule, entitled "Content and Format of Labeling for Human Prescription Drug and Biological Products; Requirements for Pregnancy and Lactation Labeling."[1]

- The final rule took effect in 2015, retiring the use of the FDA Pregnancy Risk rating categories of A, B, C, D, and X from all human prescription drug and biological product labeling. An exception to this final rule is that the new labeling system does not apply to nonprescription drugs—nonprescription drugs still utilize the Pregnancy Risk rating categories (Table 1).

- The Pregnancy Risk categories were controversial and viewed as confusing and overly simplistic. A major criticism was that they did not provide enough information for health care providers to perform a true risk-benefit assessment in collaboration with patients. The risk categories were replaced with a new

TABLE 1. U.S. FDA pregnancy risk category definitions[2]

A	Adequate and well-controlled studies in pregnant women have failed to demonstrate a risk to the fetus in the first trimester (and there is no evidence of a risk in later trimesters). Animal reproduction studies may also be available, and they fail to demonstrate a risk to the fetus.
B	Animal reproduction studies have failed to demonstrate a risk to the fetus, and there are no adequate and well-controlled studies in pregnant women, or animal reproduction studies have shown an adverse effect (other than a decrease in fertility), but adequate and well-controlled studies in pregnant women have failed to demonstrate a risk to the fetus during the first trimester of pregnancy (and there is no evidence of a risk in later trimesters).
C	Animal reproduction studies have shown an adverse effect on the fetus, there are no adequate and well-controlled studies in humans, and the benefits from the use of the drug in pregnant women may be acceptable despite its potential risks, or there are no animal reproduction studies and no adequate and well-controlled studies in humans.
D	There is positive evidence of human fetal risk based on adverse reaction data from investigational or marketing experience or studies in humans, but the potential benefits from the use of the drug in pregnant women may be acceptable despite its potential risks.
X	Studies in animals or humans have demonstrated fetal abnormalities, or there is positive evidence of fetal risk based on adverse reaction reports from investigational or marketing experience, or both, and the risk of the use of the drug in a pregnant woman clearly outweighs any possible benefit.

labeling system that is intended to provide more useful information that can effectively communicate the risk a drug may have to mother, fetus, and breastfed infants so that health care providers in collaboration with patients can make better-informed decisions.

- In evaluating the use and safety of nonprescription drugs during pregnancy, health care providers should be familiar with the A, B, C, D, X rating system and other resources for the use of drugs during pregnancy and lactation.

- Additional resources on the use of drugs in pregnancy and their FDA pregnancy risk categories can be found in the following:
    - Briggs GG, Freeman RK, Towers CV, Forinash AB. *Drugs in Pregnancy and Lactation: A Reference Guide to Fetal and Neonatal Risk.* 11th ed. Philadelphia, PA: Wolters Kluwer Health; 2017.
    - Micromedex. Truven Health Analytics, Greenwood Village, CO. http://www.micromedexsolutions.com
    - Lexi-Drugs. Lexicomp, Wolters Kluwer Health, Inc., Riverwoods, IL. http://online.lexi.com

■ ■ References

1. U.S. Food and Drug Administration (FDA). Content and format of labeling for human prescription drug and biological products; requirements for pregnancy and lactation labeling. *Fed Regist.* 2014;79(233):72063–72103.

2. U.S. Food and Drug Administration (FDA). Content and format of labeling for human prescription drug and biological products; requirements for pregnancy and lactation labeling. *Fed Regist.* 2008;73(104):30831–30868.

Recommended Intakes for Vitamins And Minerals

Nabila Ahmed-Sarwar, PharmD, BCPS, BCACP, CDE, BC-ADM

The values included in this appendix represent recommended dietary allowances (RDAs) in **bold type** and adequate intakes (AIs) in regular type followed by a single asterisk (*). Both RDAs and AIs may be used as goals for developing patient-specific recommendations.

TABLE 1. Dietary reference intakes (DRIs): RDAs and AIs, vitamins (Food and Nutrition Board, Institutes of Medicine, National Academies)

Life Stage Group	Vitamin A (µg/day)[a]	Thiamin (B₁) (mg/day)	Riboflavin (B₂) (mg/day)	Pyridoxine (B₆) (mg/day)	Biotin (B₇) (µg/day)	Cyanocobalamin (B₁₂) (µg/day)
Infants						
0–6 mo	400*	0.2*	0.3*	0.1*	5*	0.4*
6–12 mo	500*	0.3*	0.4*	0.3*	6*	0.5*
Children						
1–3 y	300	0.5	0.5	0.5	8*	0.9
4–8 y	400	0.6	0.6	0.6	12*	1.2
Males						
9–13 y	600	0.9	0.9	1.0	20*	1.8
14–18 y	900	1.2	1.3	1.3	25*	2.4
19–50 y	900	1.2	1.3	1.3	30*	2.4
51–70 y	900	1.2	1.3	1.7	30*	2.4
>70 y	900	1.2	1.3	1.7	30*	2.4
Females						
9–13 y	600	0.9	0.9	1.0	20*	1.8
14–18 y	700	1.0	1.0	1.2	25*	2.4
19–50 y	700	1.1	1.1	1.3	30*	2.4
51–70 y	700	1.1	1.1	1.5	30*	2.4
>70 y	700	1.1	1.1	1.5	30*	2.4
Pregnancy						
14–18 y	750	1.4	1.4	1.9	30*	2.6
19–50 y	770	1.4	1.4	1.9	30*	2.6
Lactation						
14–18 y	1200	1.4	1.6	2.0	35*	2.8
19–50 y	1300	1.4	1.6	2.0	35*	2.8

Source: Reprinted with permission.[1,2]
[a]As retinol activity equivalents (RAEs). 1 RAE = retinol 1 mcg, beta carotene 12 mcg, alpha carotene 24 mcg, or beta cryptoxanthin 24 mcg.
[b]Cholecalciferol 1 mcg = vitamin D 40 IU.
[c]As alpha tocopherol.
[d]As niacin equivalents (NE). Niacin 1 mg = tryptophan 60 mg; 0-6 months = preformed niacin (not NE).
[e]As dietary folate equivalents (DFE). 1 DFE = food folate 1 mcg = folic acid 0.6 mcg from fortified food or as a supplement consumed with food = supplement 0.5 mcg taken on an empty stomach.
[f]Folate intake is linked with neural tube defects in the fetus; all women capable of becoming pregnant should consume folate 400 mcg until their pregnancy is confirmed and they enter prenatal care, which ordinarily occurs after the end of the periconceptional period, the critical time for formation of the neural tube.

Vitamin C (mg/day)	Vitamin D (IU/day)[b]	Vitamin E (mg/day)[c]	Vitamin K (µg/day)	Niacin (mg/day)[d]	Folate (µg/day)[e]	Choline (mg/day)
40*	400	4*	2.0*	2*	65*	125*
50*	400	5*	2.5*	4*	80*	150*
15	600	6	30*	6	150	200*
25	600	7	55*	8	200	250*
45	600	11	60*	12	300	375*
75	600	15	75*	16	400	550*
90	600	15	120*	16	400	550*
90	600	15	120*	16	400	550*
90	800	15	120*	16	400	550*
45	600	11	60*	12	300	375*
65	600	15	75*	14	400[f]	400*
75	600	15	90*	14	400[f]	425*
75	600	15	90*	14	400[f]	425*
75	800	15	90*	14	400[f]	425*
80	600	15	75*	18	600[f]	450*
85	600	15	90*	18	600[f]	450*
115	600	19	75*	17	500	550*
120	600	19	90*	17	500	550*

TABLE 2. DRIs: RDAs and AIs, select elements (Food and Nutrition Board, Institute of Medicine, National Academies)

Life Stage Group	Calcium (mg/day)	Chromium (µg/day)	Fluoride (mg/day)	Iodine (µg/day)	Iron (mg/day)
Infants					
0–6 mo	200*	0.2*	0.01*	110*	0.27*
6–12 mo	260*	5.5*	0.5*	130*	11
Children					
1–3 y	700	11*	0.7*	90	7
4–8 y	1000	15*	1*	90	10
Males					
9–13 y	1300	25*	2*	120	8
14–18 y	1300	35*	3*	150	11
19–30 y	1000	35*	4*	150	8
31–50 y	1000	35*	4*	150	8
51–70 y	1000	30*	4*	150	8
>70 y	1200	30*	4*	150	8
Females					
9–13 y	1300	21*	2*	120	8
14–18 y	1300	24*	3*	150	15
19–30 y	1000	25*	3*	150	18
31–50 y	1000	25*	3*	150	18
51–>70 y	1200	20*	3*	150	8
Pregnancy					
14–18 y	1300*	29*	3*	220	27
19–30 y	1000*	30*	3*	220	27
31–50 y	1000*	30*	3*	220	27
Lactation					
14–18 y	1300*	44*	3*	290	10
19–30 y	1000*	45*	3*	290	9
31–50 y	1000*	45*	3*	290	9

Source: Reprinted with permission.[1,2]

■ ● References

1. National Agricultural Library, United States Department of Agriculture. DRI tables and application reports. https://www.nal.usda.gov/fnic/dri-tables-and-application-reports. Accessed July 19, 2018.

2. Institute of Medicine. *Dietary Reference Intakes for Calcium and Vitamin D*. Washington, DC: The National Academies Press; 2011.

Magnesium (mg/day)	Phosphorus (mg/day)	Selenium (µg/day)	Zinc (mg/day)
30*	100*	15*	2*
75*	275*	20*	3
80	460	20	3
130	500	30	5
240	1250	40	8
410	1250	55	11
400	700	55	11
420	700	55	11
420	700	55	11
420	700	55	11
240	1250	40	8
360	1250	55	9
310	700	55	8
320	700	55	8
320	700	55	8
400	1250	60	12
350	700	60	11
360	700	60	11
360	1250	70	13
310	700	70	12
320	700	70	12

APPENDIX 5

Common Uses for Popular Natural Products

Miranda Wilhelm, PharmD

For complete information about this topic, consult Chapter 51, "Natural Products," written by Cydney E. McQueen and Katherine Kelly Orr and published in the *Handbook of Nonprescription Drugs*, 19th Edition.[1]

The products discussed were chosen because they have evidence to support their use, are widely promoted either with or without evidence supporting use, or present known or theoretical safety concerns.

System	Natural Product	Therapeutic Uses	Dosage	Safety, Efficacy Considerations
Cardiovascular system	CoQ10	Cardiovascular conditions (e.g., heart failure, cardiomyopathy, hypertension)	100 mg by mouth 2–3 times daily with meals	Avoid in pregnancy and lactation because of lack of safety information; possible vitamin K–like procoagulant effects if taken with warfarin; monitor international normalized ratio (INR)
		Migraine prevention	300 mg by mouth daily for adults	
		Reduction of statin-associated adverse effects	50–100 mg by mouth daily	
	Fish oil	Lower triglycerides	2–4 g by mouth daily in divided doses	Possible additive effects, primarily at dosages >4 g/d if taken with anti-thrombotic agents
	Garlic	Hyperlipidemic; hypertension	Powdered garlic standardized to allicin content of 1%–1.6% (3–5 mg by mouth daily); aged garlic extract containing at least 1.2 mg S-allyl cysteine	Interaction with warfarin—increased INR; interaction with saquinavir—50% reduction in levels; interaction with oral contraceptives—decreased effectiveness; contradictory evidence regarding induction of drugs metabolized through CYP3A4 and CYP2D6; may inhibit isoniazid absorption
	Green coffee bean extract	Hypertension	140 mg chlorogenic acids by mouth daily	Possible additive effects with other antihypertensive agents; possible decreased absorption of alendronate
		Weight loss	Limited efficacy data at this time; no recommendations for weight loss can be made	
	Red yeast rice	Hyperlipidemia	1.2–2.4 g by mouth daily in 2 divided doses	Contraindicated during pregnancy; additive effect when used with statins; CYP3A4 inhibitors—possible increased levels and adverse effects; gemfibrozil—possible increased adverse effects
	Resveratrol	Hyperlipidemia	Optimal dosage has not been determined; 8–1000 mg by mouth daily may be appropriate	Headache is the most common adverse effect.

Central nervous system (CNS)	Butterbur	Allergic rhinitis	Standardized petasin 8–16 mg by mouth 3–4 times daily	Contraindicated in patients allergic to ragweed or chrysanthemums; avoid during pregnancy and lactation because of hepatotoxicity; possible interaction with anticholinergic drugs or antimigraine medications; avoid with known inducers of CYP3A4; possible pyrrolizidine increase
		Migraine prevention	Standardized extracts containing 7.5 mg petasin and 7.5 mg isopetasin per 50 mg tablet or capsule with a dose of 50–75 mg by mouth twice daily	
	Feverfew	Migraine prevention	50–100 mg by mouth daily in divided doses	Contraindicated in patients allergic to ragweed or chrysanthemums; avoid during pregnancy and lactation; possible additive effects if taken with other antithrombotic agents or herbs; possible inhibition of CYP1A2, CYP2C8, CYP2C9, CYP2C19, CYP2D6, and CYP3A4
	Ginkgo	Attention deficit hyperactivity disorder; dementia; intermittent claudication	120–240 mg by mouth daily of ginkgo leaf extract in 2–3 divided doses	Avoid in pregnancy and lactation because of lack of safety information; interaction with antithrombotic agents—possible additive effect; interaction with atorvastatin—decreased clearance; interaction with efavirenz—decreased levels; interaction with omeprazole—decreased levels; interaction with trazodone—case report of coma with low-dose trazodone; excessive ingestion associated with seizures; avoid in patients with a history of seizures or current drugs that may lower seizure threshold; potential additive effects with antihypertensive drugs, although paradoxical hypertension has been reported with hydrochlorothiazide; possible increase in levels of nifedipine; possible reduction in concentrations of ritonavir, lansoprazole, and tolbutamide
	Kava	Insomnia; mild anxiety	Avoid recommending, as kava may be associated with severe liver injury	
	Melatonin	Insomnia	0.3–5 mg by mouth daily taken 30–60 min prior to bedtime	Avoid in pregnancy and lactation; interaction with nifedipine—reduced delivery via the gastrointestinal (GI) therapeutic system; interaction with fluvoxamine, monoamine oxidase inhibitors (MAOIs), and tricyclic antidepressants—increase melatonin; interaction with benzodiazepines, sodium valproate, and beta blockers—decrease melatonin nighttime levels; caffeine or oral contraceptive use have various effects on melatonin levels; verapamil may decrease melatonin levels; possible interaction with immunosuppressant drugs related to immunostimulating properties
		Jet lag	2–5 mg by mouth in the evening the day of arrival and at bedtime for the following 2–5 d	

(continued)

System	Natural Product	Therapeutic Uses	Dosage	Safety, Efficacy Considerations
	St. John's wort	Depression	900–1800 mg by mouth daily (standardized extract of 0.3% hypericin or 2%–5% hyperforin) in 3 divided doses with meals	Avoid in pregnancy and lactation because of lack of safety information; interaction with CYP3A4 substrates—significantly decreased drug levels and effects (e.g., alprazolam, amitriptyline, atorvastatin, erythromycin, finasteride, imatinib, irinotecan, methadone, nifedipine, simvastatin, tacrolimus, verapamil, voriconazole, warfarin, zolpidem); interaction with antidepressants—increased risk of serotonin syndrome; interaction with cyclosporine—decreased blood levels of immunosuppressant, leading to transplant graft rejection; interaction with oral contraceptives and hormone therapy—decreased hormone levels, risking contraceptive failure; interaction with protease inhibitors, nonnucleoside reverse transcriptase inhibitors, and nonstructural protein 5A or 5B inhibitors—decreased serum levels; possible increased risk of serotonin syndrome if taken with 5-HT1 agonists, dextromethorphan, meperidine, and tramadol; digoxin—decreased intestinal absorption, decreased digoxin levels; possible decreased levels and effect of amiodarone, theophylline, and proton pump inhibitors; monitoring for fexofenadine toxicity recommended if taken concomitantly; morphine—increased narcotic-induced sleep time in animal studies; use with other photosensitizing agents contraindicated
	Valerian	Insomnia	400–900 mg by mouth daily administered 30–120 min before bedtime	Avoid in pregnancy because of potential for induction of uterine contractions; possible increased sedative effect if taken with alcohol or other CNS depressants; possible inhibitor of CYP3A4
Digestive system	Ginger	Nausea and vomiting in pregnancy (i.e., morning sickness)	Dried ginger 250 mg by mouth 4 times daily	Interaction with antithrombotic agents—possible additive effect; interaction with nifedipine—decreased platelet aggregation; avoid with antihyperglycemic drugs because of additive effects
		Nausea and vomiting associated with motion sickness	Dried powdered ginger 500 mg taken 30 min before travel, followed by 500–1000 mg by mouth every 4 h as needed (not to exceed 4 g daily)	

	Milk thistle	Cirrhosis Hepatitis	150 mg silymarin by mouth 3 times daily 240 mg silybin by mouth twice daily	Avoid in pregnancy and lactation because of lack of safety information; contraindicated in patients allergic to ragweed or chrysanthemums; inhibition of CYP2C9, CYP2D6, and CYP3A4 is unlikely; evidence is contradictory
	Peppermint	Irritable bowel syndrome	Enteric-coated capsules containing 0.2–0.4 mL (187–374 mg) oil by mouth 3 times daily 15–30 min before meals	Decreased absorption of iron salts; interaction with drugs that increase gastric pH—premature dissolution of enteric-coated peppermint oil capsules; possible inhibition of CYP3A4
Endocrine system	Alpha-lipoic acid	Diabetic peripheral neuropathy	600 mg by mouth 3 times daily on an empty stomach to improve absorption	Increased bioavailability of valproate; monitor blood glucose in patients taking antihyperglycemic drugs; potential chelating activity with minerals and antacids, separate by 2–3 h; possible interference with conversion of thyroxine to triiodothyronine; possible reduction of effectiveness of some chemotherapy agents
	Cinnamon	Lower blood glucose	0.5–1 g by mouth daily of aqueous extract; 2–6 g by mouth daily in divided doses of ground cinnamon	Additive effects with antihyperglycemic agents
Immune modulators	Echinacea	Prevent and treat colds	Optimal standardization and dosage have not been determined	Contraindicated in patients allergic to ragweed or chrysanthemums; possible interaction with immunomodulating therapies. CYP3A4 substrates with low oral bioavailability: verapamil, cyclosporine, tacrolimus. Effects on CYP1A2, CYP2C9, or CYP3A4 are likely to be clinically insignificant. If utilized, all formulations must be taken at the first sign of illness.
	Elderberry	Prevent and treat influenza	Optimal standardization and dosage forms have not been determined; 4 dosage forms have been studied: spray-dried juice (400 mg by mouth 3 times daily), syrup (Sambucol) 3.8 g (10 mL) by mouth daily,[2] encapsulated extract (125 mg), and dried infusion prepared daily	Possible additive effects with antihypertensive and antihyperglycemic agents; increase monitoring
Kidney, urinary tract, and prostate	African plum	Benign prostatic hyperplasia (BPH)	50–100 mg by mouth twice daily containing standardized 14% triterpenes and 0.5% n-docosanol	Potential risk for increased adverse effects when combined with finasteride or dutasteride
	Cranberry	Prevent urinary tract infections	300–900 mL by mouth daily of cranberry juice (not cranberry juice cocktail); 400 mg by mouth twice daily of capsule formulations	Possible increased INR and risk of bleeding in patients taking warfarin; possible CYP2C9 inhibition; may alter excretion of weakly alkaline drugs or neutralize effects of antacids

(continued)

System	Natural Product	Therapeutic Uses	Dosage	Safety, Efficacy Considerations
	Dehydroepiandrosterone	Enhance athletic performance or increase muscle mass; reduce physical and mental symptoms of aging; improve sexual dysfunction or sexual performance	25–100 mg by mouth daily	Avoid in pregnancy and lactation; because of risk of adverse effects, dosages greater than 25 mg per day should be used only under the guidance of a health care provider; interaction with triazolam—increased triazolam levels; interaction with antidepressants—increased risk of mania; interference with hormonal or antihormonal therapies; may increase risk of thromboembolism with oral contraceptives; possible increased levels of CYP3A4 substrates
	Saw palmetto	BPH	160 mg by mouth twice daily or 320 mg by mouth once daily	Contraindicated in pregnancy and lactation; potential interaction with hormonal or antihormonal therapy in men and women; possible additive effects when used with antithrombotic agents
Musculoskeletal system	Glucosamine, chondroitin	Osteoarthritis	1500 mg of glucosamine sulfate and 1200 mg of chondroitin sulfate by mouth daily, either once or in divided doses, with food if GI upset occurs	Avoid glucosamine in patients with shellfish allergy (use chondroitin monotherapy); avoid in pregnancy and lactation because of lack of safety information; interaction with warfarin—increased bleeding risk in individuals with variant CYP2C9 alleles; monitor blood glucose for first few days in patients taking antihyperglycemic drugs
	Kratom	Pain	Avoid recommending, as kratom is highly addictive and use can result in death	
	Methylsulfonylmethane	Osteoarthritis	1500–3000 mg by mouth daily in 1 or divided doses (not to exceed 3000 mg daily)	Avoid in pregnancy and lactation because of lack of safety information
	S-adenosyl-L-methionine	Depression Osteoarthritis	1200–1600 mg by mouth daily 400–800 mg daily in divided doses (not to exceed 800 mg daily)	Avoid in pregnancy and lactation because of lack of safety information; interaction with antidepressants and 5-HT1 agonists—increased risk of serotonin syndrome; risk of additive adverse effects with MAOIs; avoid concomitant use with corticosteroids because of possible effects on glucocorticoid concentrations
	Turmeric, curcumin	Arthritis	Optimal dosage has not been determined; 1000–1500 mg by mouth daily in divided doses may be appropriate	Interaction with sulfasalazine—significantly increased sulfasalazine levels; possible increased effects with antithrombotic agents; possible P-glycoprotein inhibition

Physical and mental performance enhancers	Asian ginseng (Panax ginseng)	Improve mental and physical stress	200 by mouth daily in divided doses of 4% standardized ginsenosides; 2–3 g by mouth daily of powdered root	Avoid in pregnancy and lactation because of lack of safety information and concern about estrogenic effects; possible additive effects with antihyperglycemic agents; monitor blood glucose; interaction with phenelzine—possible headache, tremor, and mania in case report; interaction with imatinib—increased toxicity; unpredictable effects on concurrent antithrombotic agents; possible interference with antipsychotics and immunosuppressants; possible inhibition of CYP1A1, CYP2D6, and CYP3A4
	Eleuthero (Siberian ginseng)	Improve athletic performance	300–400 mg by mouth daily of standardized eleuthero-side B or E, or both; 10 mL by mouth 3 times daily of 33% ethanolic extract	Avoid in pregnancy and lactation because of lack of safety information; after 2 mo of daily use, discontinue product for a minimum of 2 wk; interaction with digoxin—possible false elevation in digoxin plasma levels (assay dependent); interaction with caffeine—increased CNS stimulation; monitor blood glucose in patients taking antihyperglycemic drugs. Possible inhibition of CYP1A2, CYP2C9, CYP3A4 and CYP2D6; possible inhibition of P-glycoprotein; possible additive effects with antithrombotic agents
	Green tea	Performance enhancer	3–5 cups by mouth daily up to 1200 mL daily including a minimum of 250 mg of catechins daily	Avoid in pregnancy and lactation because of potential for reduced folic acid levels; additive stimulant effects with decongestants; possible antagonism of warfarin's effect; possible antagonism of concurrent sedatives related to caffeine content; possible reduction in serum folate levels
Skin conditions	Aloe vera	Wound healing (e.g., cuts, scrapes, and minor burns)	Apply a thin layer topically to affected area(s) 2–3 times daily	Avoid oral aloe as safety data are lacking
	Tea tree oil	Antiinfective	Apply thin layer of 0.4%–100% topically to affected area(s) once or twice daily	Do not swallow, as ingesting may cause confusion, ataxia, and systemic contact dermatitis
		Acne	Apply thin layer of 5% topically to affected area(s) daily	
		Athlete's foot	Apply thin layer of 25%–50% topically to affected area(s) twice daily for 4 wk	
		Fungal toenail infection	Apply thin layer of 100% topically to affected area(s) twice daily for 6 mo	

(continued)

System	Natural Product	Therapeutic Uses	Dosage	Safety, Efficacy Considerations
Weight loss	*Garcinia cambogia*, hydroxycitric acid	Weight loss	Optimal dosage has not been determined; 285 mg hydroxycitric acid alone to *G cambogia* extracts containing 2800 mg hydroxycitric acid by mouth daily may be appropriate	Interaction with selective serotonin reuptake inhibitor (SSRIs)—case report of serotonin syndrome; possible additive effects with antihyperglycemic agents
	Raspberry ketone	Weight loss	Optimal dosage has not been determined	Possible additive effects with antihyperglycemic agents
Women's health	Black cohosh	Menopausal symptoms	40 mg by mouth daily in 1–2 divided doses	Avoid in pregnancy and lactation because of potential hormonal effects; possible potentiation of antihypertensive agents; may increase toxicity of doxorubicin and docetaxel; may decrease effectiveness of cisplatin; avoid with hepatotoxic drugs
	Chasteberry	Menopausal symptoms; premenstrual dysphoric disorder, premenstrual syndrome	Optimal standardization has not been determined; 20–40 mg of extract by mouth daily	Avoid in pregnancy and lactation because of lack of safety information; possible interference with hormonal therapy or oral contraceptives; possible interaction with antipsychotics, dopamine agonists and antagonists, and metoclopramide because of dopaminergic activity
	Evening primrose oil	Mastalgia	2–4 g by mouth daily	Avoid in pregnancy and lactation because of adverse pregnancy outcomes; possible additive effects if taken with other antithrombotic agents or herbs; possible increased risk of seizure with phenothiazines; potential additive effects to antihypertensives
	Fenugreek	Stimulation of breast milk production	2–3 capsules (580–610 mg per capsule) by mouth 3–4 times daily	Contraindicated in patients allergic to chickpeas; avoid in pregnancy because of oxytocic and uterine stimulant effects; possible additive effects if taken with other antithrombotic agents or herbs; possible additive effects with antihyperglycemic drugs
		Diabetes; GI conditions; hyperlipidemia	Seed powder capsules 2.5 g by mouth twice daily, seed powder 25 g by mouth daily in 2 divided doses, or defatted seeds 100 g by mouth daily in 2 divided doses	
	Phytoestrogens	Menopausal symptoms	Optimal dosage has not been determined	Avoid in patients with hormone-sensitive cancers because of lack of safety information; possible increased risk of bleeding in patients taking anti-thrombotic agents with red clover–based products

■ ■ References

1. McQueen CE, Orr KK. Natural products. In: Krinsky DL, Ferreri SP, Hemstreet BA, Hume AL, Newton GD, Rollins CJ, Tietze KJ, eds. *Handbook of Nonprescription Drugs: An Interactive Approach to Self-Care*. Washington, DC: American Pharmacists Association; 2018:957–994.

2. Sambucol. Sambucol Black Elderberry Original Syrup. https://sambucolusa.com/products/sambucol%C2%AE-original-4-fl-oz-120-ml. Accessed June 11, 2018.

Common Probiotics

Cortney M. Mospan, PharmD, BCACP, BCGP

For complete information about this topic, consult Chapter 20, "Prebiotics and Probiotics," written by Pramodini Kale-Pradhan and Sheila Wilhelm in the *Handbook of Nonprescription Drugs*, 19th Edition.[1]

All probiotic formulations are regulated as dietary supplements, which are regulated as foods, not drugs. Thus, they are not tightly regulated. Products are not evaluated for efficacy or safety by the FDA.

This appendix provides a high-level summary for the commonly available probiotic strains with evidence to support their use. It is not an exhaustive list, but it attempts to provide practitioners with quick recommendations of commercially available products with therapeutic evidence. It is necessary to recommend probiotics down to the specific strain, as different strains will confer different health benefits.

Probiotic Definition: Live microorganisms that confer a health benefit on the host when administered in adequate amounts.

Probiotic Product	Genus	Species	Strain	Therapeutic Use	Recommended Dose	Special Notes
Activia yogurt	Bifidobacterium	lactis	DN-173 010 (CNCM 1-2494)	Digestive system regulation	Consume daily as part of therapeutic lifestyle interventions	Contains 100 million CFUs/g
Align	Bifidobacterium	infantis	35624	Irritable bowel syndrome	1 (1 billion CFUs) capsule daily	Contains milk product
Bio-K+	Lactobacillus Lactobacillus Lactobacillus	acidophilus casei rhamnosus	CL1285 LBC80R CLR2	Digestive health	1–2 capsules (50 billion CFUs) daily	Contains milk product; dairy-free formulation available; available as capsules, flavored fermented milk, fermented soy, or fermented rice; stable up to 90 d when refrigerated, 5–7 d once opened if continuing to store in refrigerator; separate from antibiotics by 2 h
				Travel protection	1 capsule (30 billion CFUs) travel protection formulation daily 3–5 d before departure; 1–2 capsules daily during trip; 1 capsule daily 3–5 d after return	
				Antibiotic-associated diarrhea (prevention)	2 capsules (50 billion CFUs) daily during treatment; continue 5 d following completion of antibiotic	
				Clostridium difficile–associated diarrhea (prevention)	2 capsules (50 billion CFUs) daily during treatment; continue 5 d following completion of antibiotic	
Culturelle Health and Wellness	Lactobacillus	rhamnosus	GG	Digestive health; acute diarrhea treatment; travel protection and immune support; antibiotic-associated diarrhea prevention	1 capsule (10 billion CFUs) daily	Take for 1–2 weeks for prevention of antibiotic-associated diarrhea; best effects if started within 48 h of antibiotics

Product	Genus	Species	Strain	Use	Dosage	Notes
Culturelle Health and Wellness	Lactobacillus	rhamnosus	GG	Eczema	1 capsule (100 billion CFUs) daily for mother during pregnancy	Mother should take for 2–4 weeks before delivery, then give infant drops into mouth, into bottle, or while breastfeeding; drops only good for 60 d once opened
Culturelle Baby Grow and Thrive Probiotics and Vitamin D Drops	Lactobacillus Bifidobacterium	rhamnosus animalis	GG BB-12	Atopic dermatitis	5 drops (2.5 billion CFUs with 10 mcg Vitamin D) daily for 6 mo	Contains 10 billion CFU/93 mL bottle
DanActive yogurt	Lactobacillus Streptococcus Lactobacillus	bulgaricus thermophilus casei	Strain designations not provided	Immune system support	Consume daily as part of therapeutic lifestyle interventions	Consume with water; also includes lactase 3000 ALU
Digestive Advantage Lactose Defense Formula	BC^{30} Bacillus	coagulans	GBI-30, 6086	Digestive health and lactose intolerance	1 capsule (2 billion CFUs) daily	
Florajen Digestion	Lactobacillus Bifidobacterium Bifidobacterium	acidophilus lactis longum	Strain designations not provided	Intestinal health; maintain immune system	1 capsule (15 billion CFUs) daily for all general uses	This product should be stored in refrigerator but can be stored up to 2 weeks at room temperature; dairy-free, gluten-free, kosher, non-GMO, allergen-free; can be sprinkled on cold food or beverages
Florajen Women	Lactobacillus Lactobacillus Lactobacillus	acidophilus acidophilus rhamnosus	La-14 NCFM HN001	Helps restore vaginal pH; helps restore and retain natural balance of vaginal flora	1 capsule (15 billion CFUs) daily	This product should be stored in refrigerator but can be stored up to 2 weeks at room temperature; dairy-free, gluten-free, kosher, non-GMO, allergen-free; can be sprinkled on cold food or beverages

(continued)

Probiotic Product	Genus	Species	Strain	Therapeutic Use	Recommended Dose	Special Notes
Florajen Kids	Lactobacillus Lactobacillus Bifidobacterium Bifidobacterium	acidophilus rhamnosus lactis lactis	NCFM HN001 Bi-07 HN019	Restores balance of good bacteria; helps minimize diarrhea associated with antibiotics	1 capsule (6 billion CFUs) daily	This product should be stored in refrigerator but can be stored up to 2 weeks at room temperature; dairy-free, gluten-free, kosher, non-GMO, allergen-free; can be sprinkled on cold food or beverages
Florastor	Saccharomyces	boulardii	CNCM I-745	Traveler's diarrhea (prevention)	1–2 capsules (250 mg) daily 5 d before trip and throughout trip duration	This is a yeast product. This product should not be refrigerated.
				Antibiotic-associated diarrhea (prevention)	2 capsules (250 mg) twice daily within 3 d of antibiotic start; continue 3 d after antibiotic is finished (total 1–4 weeks)	Product contains lactose
				C. difficile recurrence prevention	2 capsules (250 mg) twice daily for 4 weeks with appropriate antibiotic	
RepHresh Pro-B	Lactobacillus Lactobacillus	rhamnosus reuteri	GR-1 RC-14	Promotion of healthy vaginal flora	1 capsule (5 billion CFUs) daily	
Nature Made Digestive Products Advanced Dual Action	Lactobacillus Bifidobacterium	plantarum lactis	299V SD-5674	Cardiovascular risk reduction; diabetes (improves FBG)	1 capsule (10 billion CFUs L. plantarum, 5 billion CFUs B. lactis) daily	Nondairy and gluten free; must take 4–16 weeks for cardiovascular benefit (BMI, waist circumference, LDL and total cholesterol lowering); must take for at least 8 weeks for FBG improvement

Product	Genus	Species	Strain	Indication	Dose	Notes
TruBiotics with Immune Support Advantage	Lactobacillus Bifidobacterium	acidophilus animalis	LA-5 BB-12	Digestive health and health metabolism; immune health; allergic rhinitis	1 capsule (2 billion CFUs) daily	Take with a meal; should take continuously (4 weeks-12 mo) for allergic rhinitis; also includes vitamin A (2500 IU), vitamin C (60 mg), and vitamin E (30 IU)
VSL #3	Lactobacillus Lactobacillus Lactobacillus Lactobacillus Bifidobacterium Bifidobacterium Bifidobacterium Streptococcus	acidophilus plantarum paracasei bulgaricus breve infantis longum thermophilus	Strain designations not provided	Irritable bowel syndrome (×8 weeks)	1 regular packet or 2–4 capsules daily for 8 weeks (900 billion CFUs)	Available via prescription; can be mixed with cold, noncarbonated beverages or food (e.g., yogurt, ice cream, applesauce); hot drinks and food risk product decomposition; should be refrigerated or stored in freezer until use (don't move back into freezer once stored in refrigerator); can be stored at room temperature for up to 2 weeks
				Pouchitis	2–4 packets or 1–2 DS packets daily for 9–12 mo (1.8 trillion CFUs)	
				Ulcerative colitis (remission)	4–8 capsules, 1–2 regular packets, or 1 DS packet daily (900 billion CFUs)	
				Ulcerative colitis (active)	8–16 capsules, 2–4 regular packets, or 1–2 DS packets daily (1.8 trillion CFUs)	

Abbreviations used: ALU, acid lactase unit; BMI, body mass index; CFU, colony forming unit; DS, double strength; FBG, fasting blood glucose; GMO, genetically modified organism; LDL, low-density lipoprotein; IU, international unit.

◼◼ **References:**

1. Kale-Pradhan P, Wilhelm S. Prebiotics and probiotics. In: Krinsky DL, Ferreri SP, Hemstreet BA, Hume AL, Newton GD, Rollins CJ, Tietze KJ, eds. *Handbook of Nonprescription Drugs: An Interactive Approach to Self-Care.* Washington, DC: American Pharmacists Association; 2017:352–365.

2. PL Detail-Document. Comparison of common probiotic products. *Pharmacist's Letter/ Prescriber's Letter.* July 2015.

3. World Gastroenterology Organisation. Probiotics and Prebiotics. http://www.world gastroenterology.org/guidelines/global-guidelines/probiotics-and-prebiotics. Accessed August 21, 2018.

4. Florajen. Our Product Line of High Potency Live Probiotics. https://www.florajen.com/ products. Accessed August 21, 2018.

5. Rumore MM. Legal and regulatory issues in self-care pharmacy practice. In: Krinsky DL, Ferreri SP, Hemstreet BA, Hume AL, Newton GD, Rollins CJ, Tietze KJ, eds. *Handbook of Nonprescription Drugs: An Interactive Approach to Self-Care.* Washington, DC: American Pharmacists Association; 2017:57–76.

6. Schiff Vitamins. Digestive Advantage Daily Probiotics Supplement. https://www.schiff vitamins.com/products/digestive-advantage-daily-probiotic#ingredientsPane. Accessed August 21, 2018.

7. Bayer HealthCare Consumer Care. TruBiotics with Immune Support Advantage. http://labeling.bayercare.com/omr/online/trubiotics_Immune_Support_Advantage.pdf. Accessed August 21, 2018.

8. Culturelle Probiotics. Probiotics & Lactobacillus GG Products. https://www.culturelle. com/products. Accessed August 21, 2018.

9. Florastor Daily Probiotic Supplement. Florastor Daily Probiotics. https://florastor.com/ products/. Accessed August 21, 2018.

10. Bio-K+. FAQ. http://www.biokplus.com/en_us/faq. Accessed August 21, 2018.

11. Nature Made Digestive Probiotics. Our Probiotics Products. http://www.probiotics. naturemade.com/our-products.html#yjtCbkfWMIA3ksCR.97. Accessed August 21, 2018.

12. Alfasigma. VSL#3 Product Information Sheet. https://www.vsl3.com/pdf/VSL3Leaflet-PI.pdf. Accessed August 21, 2018.

Co-Editor Bios

Miranda Wilhelm, PharmD, is a clinical associate professor at Southern Illinois University Edwardsville School of Pharmacy in Edwardsville, Illinois. In addition to her faculty appointment, she is a clinical community pharmacist with Schnucks Pharmacy. She completed a postgraduate year one community pharmacy residency at B&K Prescription Shop in Salina, Kansas, affiliated with the University of Kansas School of Pharmacy.

Cortney M. Mospan, PharmD, BCACP, BCGP is an assistant professor of pharmacy at Wingate University Levine College of Health Sciences in Wingate, North Carolina. She also serves as a clinical pharmacist with Dilworth Drug & Wellness Center. She completed a community care pharmacy practice residency at The Ohio State University with practice sites at Uptown Pharmacy and the Ohio Pharmacists Association.